T0249223

❧ Praise for *Being Healthy with Yin Yoga*

"Once again, Stefanie Arend brings her wisdom to the practice of Yin Yoga. The skill in which she compassionately guides students toward the depth of their uniqueness is a reflection of her many years of dedicated practice and study."

—**TRACEE STANLEY,** owner of Pranamaya Yoga Media

"Stefanie's book is a wonderful, non-reductive manual and map of the Chinese energetic system and how Yin Yoga can support health and thriving. It will help guide you to a deeper understanding of your own inner terrain, whereupon your own wisdom will then serve as your reliable guide."

—**JOSH SUMMERS,** Yin Yoga and meditation teacher and trainer and host of the *Everyday Sublime* podcast

"I am so appreciative of Stefanie's well-thought sequences for different health conditions. Finally, an easy, go-to book for the layman who seeks to practice in the comfort of the home without being led by a teacher in class. This book outlines the purpose of each pose alongside easy-to-follow illustrations."

—**JO PHEE,** Assistant to Paul Grilley and Senior Yin Yoga Teacher Trainer

"Stefanie Arend has created a comprehensive and inspiring guide for yoga teachers and practitioners alike. In these pages, she offers us the fruit of her years of study and practice, combined with her own personal perspective; this book is a brilliant merger of traditional wisdom with contemporary approach and insight. She is making a real offering to the yoga community, providing practical tools and inspiration for the path that embraces yoga and energetics in an accessible and easy way to understand. It is a pleasure to have all of this information in one place."

SEBASTIAN & MURIELLE PUCELLE, Assistants to Paul Grilley and Senior Yin Yoga Teacher Trainers

"Stefanie's work is remarkable for many reasons: it showcases a solid and widespread knowledge of Yin Yoga, fascia, Traditional Chinese Medicine, and much more. It reveals deep wisdom on how to weave this knowledge with sensitivity and compassion to help us recover and heal. More than anything, it applies this wisdom to offer practical, nourishing, and regenerating practices accessible to everyone. I am sure this book can sustain and help many through their self-healing processes. Impressive."

ANAT GEIGER, Assistant to Paul Grilley and Senior Yin Yoga Teacher Trainer

Stefanie Arend

Be Healthy with
Yin Yoga

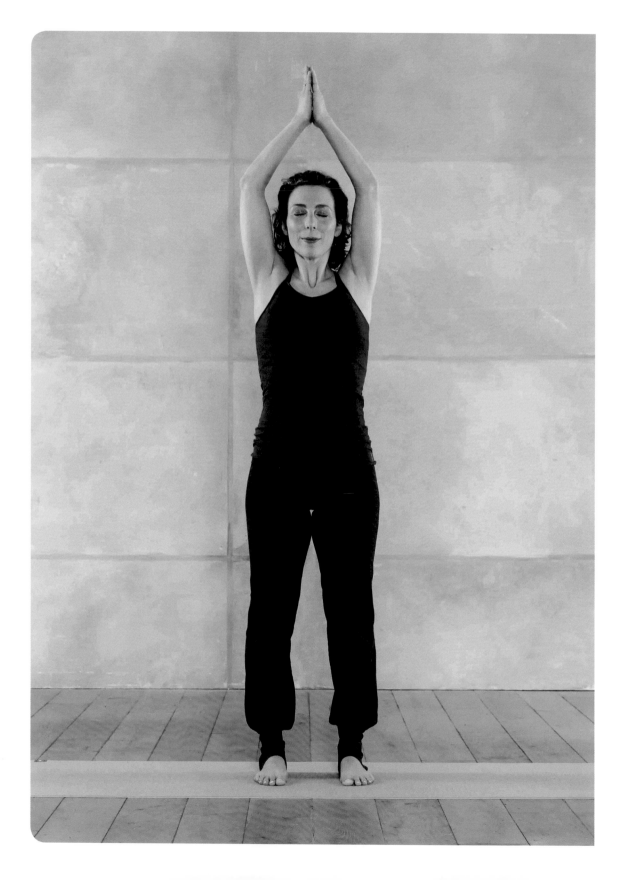

Stefanie Arend

Be Healthy with Yin Yoga

The Gentle Way to

Free Your Body of

Everyday Ailments

and Emotional Stresses

SHE WRITES PRESS

*I dedicate this book to all those who
put their trust in their capacity for self-healing
and who wish to achieve long-term health.*

*You carry your healing powers within you at all times,
but sometimes they are hidden by a lack of contact with your
inner self. A doctor, therapist, or teacher can support you
in accessing them once again—but they can only open the
door—you always have to pass through it yourself!*

Copyright © 2019 by Stefanie Arend

All rights reserved. No part of this publication may be reproduced, distributed, or transmitted in any form or by any means, including photocopying, recording, digital scanning, or other electronic or mechanical methods, without the prior written permission of the publisher, except in the case of brief quotations embodied in critical reviews and certain other noncommercial uses permitted by copyright law. For permission requests, please address She Writes Press.

Published August 2019
Printed in Canada
Print ISBN: 978-1-63152-590-2
E-ISBN: 978-1-63152-591-9
Library of Congress Control Number: 2019938513

For information, address:
She Writes Press
1569 Solano Ave #546
Berkeley, CA 94707

Interior formatting by Tabitha Lahr
Photography by Forster & Martin Fotografie, Munich

She Writes Press is a division of SparkPoint Studio, LLC.

This book is not intended as a substitute for the medical advice of physicians. The reader should regularly consult a physician in matters relating to his/her health and particularly with respect to any symptoms that may require diagnosis or medical attention. Neither the author nor the publisher are responsible for any injuries which may result from the practice of the exercises in this book.

❧ Contents

1 YIN YOGA IN THEORY

2 YIN YOGA IN PRACTICE

3 YIN YOGA FOR HEALTH AND WELL-BEING

❦ Foreword by **Paul Grilley**

Who needs theories?

Running makes us feel good, weight lifting makes us feel good, cycling makes us feel good, and hatha yoga makes us feel good. All of these forms of exercise make us feel good, and most of us don't need a chemical or physiological explanation of how that happens. But a theory of yoga can make a difference in how we practice and what we experience. Yoga has an external aspect that makes it similar to other forms of exercise, but yoga also has an internal aspect that leads us to emotional and mental insights.

The connecting thread from external to internal, from Yang to Yin, is the movement of energy in our body. Focusing on how this energy moves draws our awareness inward. Having a theory of how this happens is very helpful. This theory is provided in the textbooks of Chinese medicine, particularly acupuncture theory. There are two foundational theories of acupuncture. First, there is a life force called *Chi*. Second, this life force circulates through channels called *meridians*.

Chi is called a life force because it intelligently adapts the activities of the body's cells to resist disruptive forces that are constantly striving to create imbalance and illness. Without Chi, our bodies would decompose into a putrid pool of chemicals, which is what happens at death. Chi circulates through meridians that have been described in greater and sometimes lesser detail since ancient times. One of the modern objections to acupuncture in general and meridians in particular is that dissections have never found the meridians that are illustrated in acupuncture textbooks. This is why the modern theories of *fascia* are important.

Fascia physiology makes it plausible that meridians are electrically conductive channels of water in our fascia. This fascia/meridian theory has been demonstrated in several experiments by my own teacher, Dr. Hirioshi Motoyama. This fascia/meridian theory makes it perfectly clear why hatha yoga developed as a unique system of stretching and joint manipulation. Stretching and joint manipulation stimulates the fascia and, therefore, the flow of Chi through the meridians.

The more difficult scientific hurdle is establishing the existence of Chi. Does Chi exist? How is it different from chemical or electrical energy? This is not the place for a long discussion of the evidence, but we can use it as a jumping-off point to a discussion of objective and subjective experience.

Materialists assert that our emotions and thoughts are only electrical/chemical reactions in the brain. This is the great divide: science can only objectively study electrical/chemical reactions, but we never *subjectively experience* these things. We subjectively experience thoughts and emotions, peace and aggravation, desire and contentment.

I have the greatest respect for the scientific process, but science moves slowly. We need to be cautious when making claims about Chi and meridians and yoga. We need to have the scientific humility to recognize that our theories may be mostly right or all wrong. It will take many years of patient research before science has thoroughly tested the ancient theories of Chi and meridians.

The objective evidence for Chi and meridians will take years to develop, but the subjective evidence can be explored every day by every practicing yogini. Each day, each yogini can test to see if Yin Yoga makes her calmer, more content, and more healthy. Each day, each yogini can test to see if there is a connection between her liver and her eyes, or between stress and her lower back, or between worrying and her digestion.

Yin Yoga is ideally suited to assist in these subjective experiments. Yin Yoga stresses the fascial meridians with long, gentle poses and then gives us time to relax and feel the rebound of Chi after each pose. Little by little, the energetic connections become perceptible, and little by little we become aware of the connections between our thoughts, our emotions, and our Chi.

Stefanie's book is a great introduction to Yin Yoga. She outlines meridian theory, and then outlines specific routines. After each routine she suggests what inner behaviors to reflect upon and explains the relevant traditional Chinese medical theories. I believe this book will help aspiring yoginis systematically explore their mind-body interconnection.

Paul Grilley, founder of Yin Yoga and author of *Yin Yoga: Outline of a Quiet Practice* and *Yin Yoga: Principles and Practice*

Watsonville, California
2017

❦ Foreword by **Dr. Angela Montenegro**

Traditional Chinese Medicine teaches us that there is no Yang without sufficient Yin, and vice versa. Yang stands for activity and energy, and Yin for balancing and strengthening calmness. It is only when the Yin base is powerful enough and the Yang nourishes that the strength of Yang can have any effect.

Nowadays we live in an age that emphasizes Yang. Children have to get up early, hurry off to school, follow lessons with full concentration, and then still do their homework conscientiously. It continues with training at the sports club and/or music lessons, etc. Then there might be some time left over to play. And many adults continue this rhythm. They often make their way to work in early traffic congestion and they have to be efficient in their job, and accompanying this pressure is what they impose upon themselves. Organizing everyday matters has to happen alongside this . . . and then, perhaps, there is a bit of time remaining for fitness or well-being—keeping one eye on the clock, of course. There is often not enough time to rest—for the Yin, a focus on the self and centering yourself.

The energy of the Yin and Yang meridians circulates within all of us. These main meridians form a circulation of life energy, and every individual meridian fulfills a very specific function in this circulation; each meridian is allocated to a certain organ system and will pass through it at a given time. Yang represents activity, dynamism, and heat, and Yin stands for calm, nourishment, and cold. Neither principle cancels the other out, but they complement each other. They are opposites, but they depend on one another. And they limit each other—water limits fire, rain limits dryness, and night limits day. You are only healthy when all functional circuits of Yin and Yang are working together in harmony. If the body and mind are not rested regularly, the Yin becomes exhausted, and the Yang energy can no longer be sufficiently nourished. Then symptoms—such as lack of concentration, high blood pressure, and burnout—may result.

For this reason it is important to listen to your body and mind, to center yourself, and to strengthen the Yin. This is where Yin Yoga comes in. This form of yoga reinforces basic energy, and thereby has a positive impact on many disorders and illnesses; it also helps avoid diseases in particular. Even after a short period of regular Yin Yoga practice you will feel stronger, healthier, and more balanced.

Dr. Angela Montenegro

❧ Preface by **Stefanie Arend**

My occupation is my vocation. I am more than happy that I have been able to pass on the wonderful gift of Yin Yoga to so many people in my classes and trainings for many years. When I practice Yin Yoga, I become myself completely and experience a deep feeling of peace within myself. In Yin Yoga I am fully myself and do not have to please anyone else—either proverbially or in reality. While some types of yoga specify precisely how certain positions should look, and many of those practicing it try to emulate this ideal image, Yin Yoga is oriented towards the person practicing it. Our inner teacher is the most important yoga teacher and only considers this one individual body. I believe there is great healing potential within this as only we ourselves sense what is best for us.

I have been able to naturally gather plenty of teaching experience specifically in Yin Yoga, and as contact with people is important and I am truly interested in their feedback, I have also been lucky enough to come across and support many cases of successful regeneration. Time and again, people tell me about the positive changes they perceive since they have been practicing Yin Yoga regularly. I am delighted by this and it underlines the incredible effect of this quiet practice that directs energy, which I have so often experienced myself. These are my private studies, if I may call them that, which I would like to report precisely as they occurred.

I would not feel comfortable, however, in claiming that individual positions or sequences can cure a certain illness. A healing process is of course much more comprehensive, and even though I have been involved in health topics in depth for many years, I am nevertheless not a doctor and always consult a doctor of Traditional Chinese Medicine (TCM) whom I trust, and who is at best also a conventional medical practitioner. More and more studies show that many complaints can be alleviated, that the body can be strengthened, and that a healing journey can be supported through yoga.

You will therefore also find programs in this book that are directed specifically at individual conditions.

I am very pleased that you have chosen this book, and hope you enjoy finding out about the positive effect Yin Yoga can have on your body and well-being.

Blessings, **Stefanie Arend**

❧ Introduction

I am convinced that we have extremely good opportunities for healing with regard to many symptoms, if different therapeutic approaches are used to complement one another. If Western conventional medicine and alternative healing techniques—such as Traditional Chinese Medicine (TCM) or Ayurvedic medicine—are used together, this gives individuals more personal responsibility and a great deal can be achieved overall.

For example, I do not consider it responsible to look for a doctor just to have a medicine prescribed for current complaints and to hope that everything will be fine again—without any further questioning. Unfortunately, essential conventional medicine increasingly focuses on combating symptoms and less on looking for the cause. Also, exceedingly few doctors have the time required to concentrate intensively on the history of the individual patient. Alternative medical practitioners, on the other hand, tend to look for the origin of the complaints, and they view people holistically. Therefore, the individual patient does not enter into self-reflection in this way, for nobody can evaluate personal background and possible associations better than the person herself or himself. To do this, of course, we also require rest periods, or (for example) regular Yin Yoga practice, which directs the senses inwards and can bring us into deep contact with ourselves. The mind speaks very softly, and these periods of withdrawal are absolutely vital to understand it and find out what the body can express with symptoms. It is said that when the mind is not being listened to, the body sounds the alarm through illness, thereby making the person slow down.

In yoga books, you read about the many healing effects of individual exercises. For example, Headstand is said to supply the brain with blood, Shoulderstand has a positive effect on the thyroid gland, or Cobra activates the adrenal glands. A great deal of this has since been refuted, and I am thankful that nowadays we can find out and learn more and more about associations within the body. To give an example: with Shoulderstand and Cobra, a healing effect was assumed as it was believed that pressure on the organs had a stimulating or harmonizing effect. However, the thyroid and adrenal glands are endocrine glands, which are not affected by external pressure, and therefore these assumptions are unfortunately not true. I do not want to make such promises at all in this book. Yin Yoga has much more to do with activating energetic flow in the meridians—the energy pathways—and bringing them into harmony through individual exercises.

Besides this, it is important to relax completely in order to listen to the inner doctor and healer, who is the wisest of all.

If you learn to understand the associations of the body, then you can also assume much greater personal responsibility. I will give an example from my own experience. In the seventh grade I had to wear spectacles for the first time. This is nothing unusual in itself, but after that my vision progressively worsened a little, and when I got a driving permit, I also became aware that I was night-blind, which I found pretty disconcerting. And unfortunately, the only advice from my optician was not to drive in the dark any more, as there was nothing that could be done about night-blindness. I was not satisfied with this assertion. I had heard that acupuncture can also have a positive effect on vision and I therefore had my first experience of alternative therapies with this. My TCM doctor performed acupuncture on my liver back then, declaring that there is a connection between the liver and eyes. This was a completely new insight for me, but the needles had an effect: my vision did not improve, but it did not worsen anymore. This was reason enough for me, later on, to integrate my own liver sequence into my Yin Yoga program, which I still practice today. Since then, I only need glasses for driving. I still have to take care when driving at night, but as I am more than double the age I was back then, and my eyesight has not worsened and has even improved quite a bit, I consider this to be a superb (Yin Yoga) success.

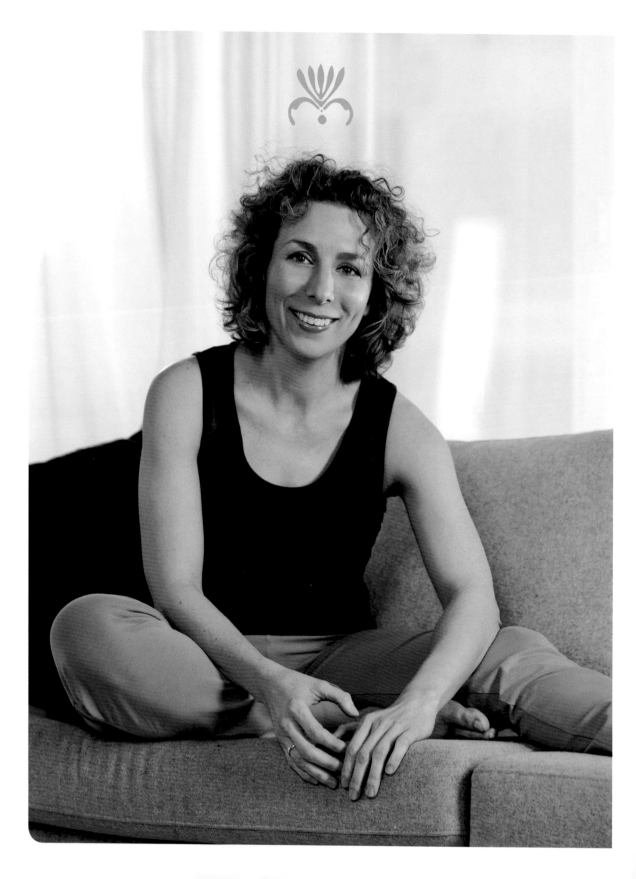

Yin Yoga in Theory

Yin Yoga is a gentle practice that harmonizes the flow of energy, and can therefore activate our capacity for self-healing. It directs us to look inwards, calms the vegetative nervous system, and relaxes and strengthens the entire body. You will find out in this chapter why Yin Yoga addresses our fascia in a targeted way, and the part played by the Chi, the meridians, and the chakras.

❧ What Is **Yin Yoga?**

As with any yoga practice, the aim of Yin Yoga is to bring the body, mind, and spirit into harmony. Based on the teaching of the Tao, each person is characterized by Yin and Yang—two opposing forces, the relationship of which should also be harmonious. Although Yin Yoga has only become very popular in the last few years, this practice also has an ancient tradition. Early writings on yoga described Yin Yoga positions, and you will also find the ancient Indian (Sanskrit) names of most exercises in this book (not including newly created ones).

My first Yin Yoga teacher was Paul Grilley, a mentor who has been a great inspiration and influence in my personal yoga practice. He made Yin Yoga into what we understand it to be today. He combined the gentle passive stretches that are held for a long time with teaching regarding the meridians, and also researched the influence of the positions upon the individual anatomy of a person.

What effect does Yin Yoga have?

Yin Yoga is an intensive and at the same time very passive practice. The exercises are carried out without any muscular tension and the breathing should also be very gentle and effortless—we simply observe it. In Yin Yoga, you hold each position for around 3 to 5 minutes and your body remains as passive as possible. The more advanced practitioners may hold each position for longer if they feel the impulse to do this, but holding it for a short time is of course also an option. These passive stretches have a positive effect on the deep layers of the body, and more particularly on the fascia. They help to loosen adhesions and shortening in the fascial structures in a gentle way and to make the tissue supple again. Yin Yoga therefore reduces pain, encourages mobility, and—not least—harmonizes the flow of energy in the meridians, as large parts of the meridians run the same course as the fascia chains in the body.

Individual Yin Yoga practice

Yoga practice should always be adapted to personal requirements, free from any performance goals. Through mindfulness and treating our own body with care, we make contact with and perceive signals from the body, which are important pointers for us. The inner yoga teacher is the most important teacher we will ever meet on a yoga journey, and it will tell you a great deal about yourself. Only it can guide you, for you alone know how a position feels deep inside.

᠅ **Fascinating Fascia** ᠅

There is a great deal of intensive research being conducted worldwide on the subject of fascia, which are the soft part of the connective tissue through which most of the meridians run. At a fascia symposium, Dr. Robert Schleip, Germany's best-known fascia researcher, made reference to longer stretches ensuring better healing of wounds in the body and reducing inflammation. It has also been found that cancer cells can spread more in rigid tissues than in well-stretched ones. The fascia that are particularly addressed by Yin Yoga practice are closely associated with our immune system. They distribute oxygen and nutrients in the body and take waste material into the bloodstream and lymph channels for excretion. With gentle but highly effective stretching and the compressions that Yin Yoga exercises exert on the body, stored toxins can be mobilized and carried away.

It is not necessary to warm up before practicing Yin Yoga, as the effect on the fascial tissues can be even more intense if you are not already sweating beforehand. The characteristic of cold is assigned to Yin, whereas Yang stands for heat. You could say that the fascia have Yin qualities, and that muscles, in turn, have Yang qualities. It is therefore reasonable to combine the relevant tissue with the relevant state. Muscles therefore respond more intensively if they are warmed up, but the opposite is true for fascia. Admittedly, the fascia can relax very well in heat, but the effect is not as lasting as if they were in a cool condition.

Of course particular care should be taken if you start your Yin Yoga practice without warming up first. It is important here that you give your body time to feel its way into the exercises. Wait patiently until it is ready to open up into the position and yield to the stretch stimuli. Tightening up the body, either on your part or because of instruction by the teacher, would be a form of external manipulation and could lead to injuries. If you take this into account, then I believe Yin Yoga is one of the styles of yoga with the lowest risk of injury, as the practice can be adapted individually to the requirements of the body.

Only go so far into a position that you feel a pleasant (!) stretch. Remain completely passive, keep your muscles relaxed, and patiently leave any other effort to gravity for the next few minutes. Indeed, you can correct your position in between, if you feel that you can achieve a more suitable stretch or if

⤞ **Practical Helpers** ⤝

Yin Yoga is a gentle form of exercise in which you should feel well and relaxed at all times. Props can therefore play an important part in the practice, and they can help you to adapt the positions to your body in the best possible way.

You should have the following props ready when you practice yoga:

- A soft base: for example, a thick yoga mat or a blanket
- A yoga bolster or a long, thick cushion
- A few yoga blocks or books
- A chair or sofa cushion or, alternatively, a rolled-up blanket
- Two small (fairly soft) balls: for example, two tennis balls.

any feeling of pain develops, but please avoid constantly fidgeting during the time you are holding it. Become internally still and watch what is happening in your body, with your breath, and in your mind over the next few minutes.

Then come out of the position slowly again. I recommend feeling your way into a neutral stomach or back position for around one minute—and, if you wish, when changing sides as well. This enables you to neutralize the body again and appreciate your energy flow, which has been activated by the exercises. Immediately after completing the positions, the energy flows through the body particularly powerfully.

I would make a distinction between *sweet pain* and *bitter pain.* Sweet pain describes a pleasant stretch stimulus that makes you feel very comfortable and at ease. This is what we wish to achieve with Yin Yoga. Bitter pain, on the other hand, goes beyond sweet pain, tends to come out selectively, and feels sharp or stabbing. You should avoid this type of pain at all costs and change the positions accordingly instead, using props or coming out of the position sooner.

✤ How Can Yin Yoga **Activate the Capacity for Self-Healing?**

Yang belongs to the Yin, and Yin belongs to the Yang. Nevertheless, I do not really want to go into the Yang components of the body too much in this book. Of course, it is still important to nourish your Yang. However, in this current age we have a surplus of Yang in our environment, which can trouble us at a physical level. Never before have there been so many hyperactive children as there are today—I tend to find the term "hyperactive" unsuitable, and I am only using it here for the ease of understanding—and "burnout" is heedlessly named as a fashionable complaint. Where has this suddenly come from? An important cause is anxiety, which can be worsened due to an excess of Yang. Think for a moment how everything has changed over the years: Barely anybody takes time out to rest in the early afternoon nowadays; due to mobile accessibility we still receive calls or text messages late in the evening when we should actually be resting; the TV is on all day in some households, even when nobody is consciously following it; there are fewer family meals; the performance mentality at school and at work is ever-present; attentive conversations without glancing at your mobile phone have also become rare. All these things exhaust our Yin. Yin and Yang are then no longer in balance, which has adverse consequences. If these energies fall out of their dynamic balance, energy can no longer flow harmoniously and this creates the circumstances for illnesses to occur.

Getting in touch

Yin Yoga practice gives us the peace that we so urgently need in this noisy world. We can use it to get in touch with our inner selves once again. Our body awareness is trained and intensified through long and deep stretches, but these also provide us with calm so that memories or emotions can emerge again. If we become our own quiet observer and look and listen carefully to what it is showing us, it is quite possible that we will even be able to trace the causes of certain complaints in time. The body communicates with us constantly, but many have forgotten how to listen to it and interpret its signs. For example, if we experienced emotional damage in childhood, this can have an effect into adult life. Symptoms often appear—such as nervousness, anxiety, depressive malaise, or sleep disturbances—which can be treated quickly with medicines, but the actual causes of the complaints remain unrecognized and untreated. It is therefore important to become aware of what is going on inside us, no matter whether it is pleasant or painful. If we identify what is causing us stress, then we can accept it, process it, and ultimately let it go. This progression can be very liberating and is a complete contrast to the repression of unpleasant experiences or memories. A repression mechanism never works in the long term. Whatever is behind it will keep occurring until it is accepted, understood, and released.

Yin Yoga practice, with its passive stretches that last for minutes, teaches us in a wonderful way about the process of letting go. If we have learned to let go physically, we can then also let go better emotionally and mentally.

Questioning the symptoms

The peaceful and introverted Yin Yoga practice gives us sufficient space to question pain or illnesses and find out what the body is trying to tell us. Popular opinion tells us that our bodies react to stress with a variety of symptoms. The following sayings, for example, allow us to draw conclusions about our individual organs or areas of the body, and we can surmise how complex the associations can be. Think about the phrases you have probably already used.

- I'm carrying the weight of the world on my shoulders.
- I'm getting it in the neck.
- That's getting on my nerves.
- My flesh is crawling.
- My blood is up.
- It takes my breath away.
- That makes my stomach turn.
- I can argue until I'm blue in the face.
- I'm sick and tired of it.
- It's freaking me out.
- I'm crapping myself.

(Re-)discovering the inner center

I have already experienced with great pain at a personal level how closely associations can manifest between the emotional and physical levels. I was traumatized when my beloved father died suddenly, very young and unexpectedly. Despite many years of practicing yoga, the pain of grief made my body become rigid and hard in just a few weeks. Although I grieved very intensively and cried a great deal, let the pain emerge, and took plenty of time out, I was deeply shaken by this experience, which completely threw me off course. It took a few weeks until I felt the impulse to take up my Yin Yoga practice again. And I felt as though I had never practiced before. My body was limited in its movements and barely allowed any stretching, and I could feel the pain everywhere, particularly in my shoulder and neck area.

With a great deal of patience, I gained access to my body again through small sets of exercises. I went through many emotional roller coaster rides, accepted them, and dealt with them so that I could go through the healing process step by step.

However, the Yin Yoga practice can have very healing effects on the body even with physical injuries or after operations. Here is another example from my personal experience. I had to undergo a stomach operation, and although I felt very well thanks to my many years of yoga practice, after this intervention I felt as though I was cut off from my body. It was as if the area around the scars was numb, and my stomach area no longer belonged to me . . . until I was finally able to take a cautious approach again with a few gentle Yin exercises, which I adapted to my current exercise practice using many props. After the first gentle stretches I sensed a rush of blood flowing through my body once again, and felt back to normal in my body. I returned to my own body more and more. The feeling of numbness slowly left me, and I felt how the healing energy began to flow through my meridians again, which had been separated due to the incisions in my stomach. Rarely had I felt so grateful for my Yin Yoga practice as in this situation—that I was able to do so much to speed up my own healing (on the condition of approval from the doctor in such cases, of course).

I would not have had these experiences in my Yang Yoga practice. Practicing it actively and powerfully would have overtaxed my body at the time, and would not have given me the time to feel so intensively and to deal with internal issues. Nevertheless, it is important not to view Yin and Yang so simplistically that you try to push yourself again, but rather to see the individual integrity within them. Therefore, the sequences and recommendations in this book are not a means of healing that is set in stone, but rather an option for the way ahead. Ultimately it is all about activating the capacity for self-healing in your own body. And YOUR path might be very different from that of your partner, your friends, or your family.

Benefit from experience

Science often lags behind when it comes to the subject of energy, and of course science cannot always prove everything. In Asia, meridian healing has been well known since ancient times, and treating the meridians for various complaints is standard practice. However, as meridians are not physically tangible and science cannot prove their existence, treatments such as acupuncture have long remained impermissible by health insurance companies. It was only when clinical studies proved the effectiveness of acupuncture treatments that health insurance companies began to assume the costs for it. However, scientific proof is not crucial for me, as I much prefer to rely on experiential reports from people with whom I work personally, where I can observe and confirm the successes. Since I am also a Yin Yoga teacher trainer, I always ask my participants for feedback, so I have received a great number of experiential reports. However, sometimes there are also messages from people I have not met before, and who send me feedback after working with my DVDs or books. It always fills me with joy and delight when I find out that Yin Yoga has helped people with every possible symptom. As yoga not only helps the muscles, the fascia, and nervous system, but also has the effect of reducing stress, releasing anxiety, and brightening your mood, this holistic practice is very versatile. For example, it can alleviate the side effects of chemotherapy and radiation therapy, and can enable cancer patients to get in touch with their body again; it can reduce the symptoms of multiple sclerosis, as well as fibromyalgia, asthma, and depression; and it can play an important part in the healing process for more everyday complaints such as backache, digestive problems, or general internal turmoil.

Since each person reacts differently, with Yin Yoga it is essentially a trial and error approach. You test what works well for the individual and what does not. This is basically just like conventional medicine: if a patient does not tolerate a medicine well (even if it has helped many other people), it does not make sense to continue with this medicine. Then you test whether another compound works better.

You can see that Yin Yoga offers many individual creative possibilities, and there are plenty of good reasons to practice regularly—even if you only find time to do it once a week. It also brings the energy flow into harmony and has a positive effect on body, mind, and soul. Sometimes even a supposedly small stimulus can have a major effect, in a similar way to classic homeopathy.

✻ A Quick **Guide to Oriental Medicine**

When Western medicine is used to treat patients, it usually concentrates upon what is visible, tangible, and measurable—basically, upon the functioning of a specific organ, individual body tissues, or specific laboratory values. This is quite different from Oriental medicine, which is enjoying increasing popularity; with its best-known representative, TCM, it has begun to complement conventional medicine in many fields. TCM views the body as a whole, and always sees the causes of complaints and illnesses as an impaired flow of the life energy of the Chi. Typical treatment patterns, such as acupuncture, special massage techniques, or even movement exercises such as Qigong and Yin Yoga, are called for here; their objective is to release Chi blockages and (re-)harmonize the flow of energy. You will find out in the paragraphs below how the energy system of the body is designed, and encounter the terms you will meet time and time again in this connection.

Yin and Yang—the contrasting pair

If you follow Traditional Chinese Medicine, then everything that exists is assigned to either Yin or Yang. For example, Yin stands for darkness, cold, and passivity, whereas Yang represents light, heat, and activity. However, the division into Yin and Yang is not a fixed principle, but is subject to change and dependent upon various factors. For example, the night is assigned to Yin and the day to Yang. The closer it comes to morning, the more Yang moves towards Yin, and the nearer the end of the day, the closer the Yin moves towards Yang. The Yin-Yang symbol (in Chinese, "Taijitu") demonstrates via the opposing dot in each sign that anything Yin also possesses some Yang, and Yang also carries some Yin. We also have divisions between Yin and Yang in the body, for the organs and meridians as well as for tissues.

Chi—energy of life

With Chi (also *Qi* in Chinese or *Prana* in Sanskrit), Chinese medicine describes the *life energy* or vital energy of our organism. In this respect we have different types of Chi. One of them is the Chi that has been passed onto us by our parents and is stored in the kidneys. This Chi can become depleted, as it cannot be renewed. Therefore, in TCM, the kidneys are also described as a treasure chest. An extreme lifestyle, incorrect nutrition, too much stress, intoxicants, or negative environmental factors can deplete the Chi in the kidneys. On the other hand, there is also renewable Chi, which we can always replace through breathing exercises, yoga, Tai-Chi, Qigong, meditation, healthy eating, sufficient sleep, fresh air, or a nourishing lifestyle.

The meridians—the energy pathways of the body

A meridian—an energy pathway, which has a physical as well as an energetic effect at the same time—can be compared to a river in which there is always movement. Nature benefits most from this river when the water flows evenly, as it waters the countryside and provides a living space for fish. However, if the river loses more and more water due to a sustained dry period, this can be as damaging to nature as a flood of water over the banks due to too much rain. This can also apply to people: the meridians run through our whole body, on the surface as well as deep inside, and they supply the organs, fascia, muscles, and every cell with life energy, the Chi. Too little energy can be just as unfavorable as too much energy. To maintain the health of the body, it is vital to keep these energies in balance and harmony so that illnesses do not arise.

Jing Mai—the twelve main meridians

There are twelve main meridians (in Chinese, "Jing Mai"), which run in a mirror image through the left and right sides of the bodies. Ten of these are associated with individual organs, and two others have a protective function and are not allocated to an organ. In addition, there are two special meridians in the center of the upper body, on the front and rear side, which are also not linked to an organ. Besides these, there are numerous cross-connections and deeper meridians that play a lesser part in Yin Yoga practice, which places emphasis on the organ meridians.

Ren Mai & Du Mai—two wonder meridians

Although the deeper meridians are less in focus in Yin Yoga, you will nevertheless encounter two of these at some point in this book: the conception (in Chinese, "Ren Mai") attributed to Yin, and the Yang-oriented governing vessel (in Chinese, "Du Mai"). They are among the eight extraordinary vessels (in Chinese, "Qi Jing Mai")—also described as the *wonder meridians*—which conserve the Chi at a deep level and can pass it on to the main meridians if required.

The chakras—the centers of energy of the body

According to Indian teaching, the chakras describe the centers of energy in the body—little round vortexes which can receive energy, concentrate it, strengthen it, and distribute it in the body. The chakras are arranged along the vertical central axis of the body and are connected to one another via lines of energy (known as "Nadis" in Sanskrit), as well as with the meridians, and in large part these lines of energy are also located within the meridians. All energy systems of the body correspond with one another.

According to chakra teaching there are seven main chakras:

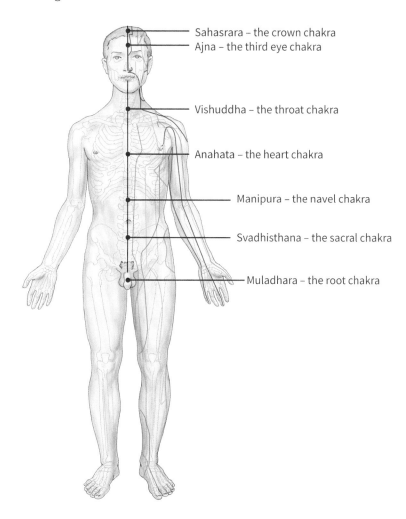

Sahasrara – the crown chakra
Ajna – the third eye chakra

Vishuddha – the throat chakra

Anahata – the heart chakra

Manipura – the navel chakra

Svadhisthana – the sacral chakra

Muladhara – the root chakra

Functional circuits—the organ system in TCM

When you look at someone stretching their arms upwards, the Yin meridians run on the front or inside from the ground towards the sky, i.e. from below to above (with the exception of the stomach meridian, which is allocated to Yang). On the other hand, the Yang meridians on the rear or outside run from the sky towards the ground, i.e. from above to below. The Yin and Yang meridians connect with one another at the toes and fingers, and thereby form a circuit. You can imagine a rice farmer at work in the field: the body areas that are turned towards the sky—i.e. the rear side or the outside— correspond with Yang, and the areas that are turned towards the ground—that is, the front side or inside—correspond with Yin.

The lung, spleen, heart, kidney, pericardium, and liver meridians belong to the Yin. The peri- cardium meridian has a protective function. A special Yin meridian on the front center of the body is the conception vessel, and is not associated with an organ. The Yin organs (in Chinese, "Zang") are described as *storage organs,* as they produce the basic substances the body requires to maintain its functions.

There is a little mnemonic for the Yang meridians, which helped me to learn them at first: they all include the vowel "a." These are the large intestine, stomach, small intestine, bladder, triple warmer, and gallbladder meridians. The triple warmer meridian has a protective function. A special Yang merid- ian on the rear center of the body is the governing vessel and is not linked with an organ. As hollow organs, the task of the Yang organs (in Chinese, "Fu") is to digest food, take in nutrients, and transport and excrete waste products.

The five elements—everything changes

The view and meaning of the organs in TCM is not comparable with the ideas of Western medicine. Yin and Yang organs are not just limited to the anatomy of each organ in itself, but also include the relevant functional cycle. At the same time, each functional cycle is represented by an element, to which the specific organs and meridians, body tissues, emotions, chakras, sensory perceptions, and colors—as well as climate conditions and seasons—can be assigned. For example, the kidneys are often associated with the notion of anxiety, and problems with the ears may hint at a disrupted energy flow in the area of the kidney meridian. As the interplay of the five elements is always a dynamic pro- cess, we also talk of the *five transformation phases.*

The following table gives a summary of the five functional circuits and the various topics of the elements.

	Wood	Fire	Earth	Metal	Water
Organs	Liver, gallbladder	Heart, small intestine	Spleen, stomach	Lungs, small intestine	Kidneys, bladder
Storage organ, Yin meridian	Liver	Heart	Spleen	Lungs	Kidneys
Hollow organ, Yang meridian	Gallbladder	Small intestine	Stomach	Large intestine	Bladder
Body Aperature	Eyes	Tongue	Mouth	Nose	Ears
Tissues	Tendons, muscles	Blood, blood vessels	Connective tissues, muscles, blood	Skin, hair	Bones, joints, teeth
Chakra	Navel chakra	Heart chakra	Navel chakra	Throat chakra	Root chakra, sacral chakra
Emotion	Anger, worry, sympathy	Hate, stress, love, joy	Concern, composure	Grief, courage	Anxiety, wisdom
Function	Controls the flow of Chi as well as the detoxifying of the body	Blood circulation, taking in nutrients	Digestion, distribution of nutrients	Breathing, excretion	Sex organs, urinary system, cleansing the blood
Color	Green	Red	Yellow	White	Blue, black
Season	Spring	Summer	Late Summer	Autumn	Winter
Climate	Windy	Hot	Moist/humid	Dry	Cold
Taste	Sour	Bitter	Sweet	Spicy	Salty

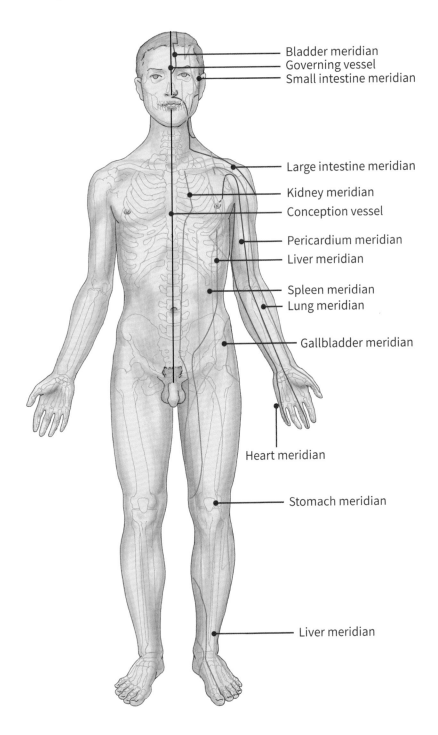

Bladder meridian
Governing vessel
Small intestine meridian

Large intestine meridian

Kidney meridian

Conception vessel

Pericardium meridian

Liver meridian

Spleen meridian
Lung meridian

Gallbladder meridian

Heart meridian

Stomach meridian

Liver meridian

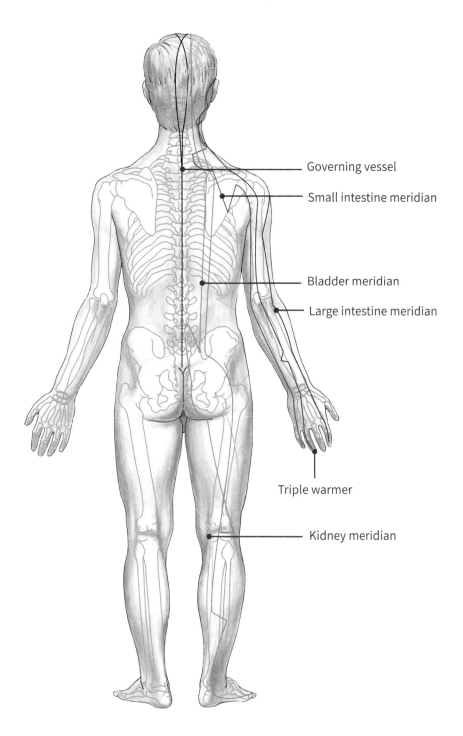

Governing vessel

Small intestine meridian

Bladder meridian

Large intestine meridian

Triple warmer

Kidney meridian

The organ clock—cycles of the Chi

Those wanting to track down tangible complaints and approach these in a targeted way would do well to turn to the so-called *organ clock*. With the two-hour change of the Chi cycle, a meridian has an energetic high point at a certain time. Within a twelve-hour period, it will reach its energetic low point, or *rest phase*.

To clarify: what is striking is that many people wake up at night between 1 and 3 a.m., and that is the time for the liver. The liver is an important organ of detoxification, and at this time it is working at full blast. If the body has to fight a great deal of toxins or acids, the liver may be overburdened—and this overload can disturb the sleep in this timespan. Most heart attacks occur between 11 a.m. and 1 p.m., in the period when the heart demonstrates the greatest activity according to the organ clock (my beloved father succumbed to a sudden cardiac failure in this very period). On the other hand, asthma attacks often strike between 3 and 5 a.m., during the maximum time for the lungs. Bowel movements work most easily in the early morning between 5 and 7 a.m., as this is the most active phase for the large intestine. The perfect time for breakfast is between 7 and 9 a.m., as the stomach is highly activated and optimally utilizes the first meal of the day. These few examples show that the organ clock can be helpful in many respects, in everyday life as well as in diagnosing the treatment of conditions.

For a TCM doctor, identifying the time factor is therefore an important key for certain conditions. They will usually ask the patient when symptoms typically arise. An excess or an abundance of Chi has an impact at the peak times of the organ clock; a lack of Chi or an empty condition, on the other hand, comes in at the rest phase twelve hours later. With these associated phases, the twelve main meridians form the so-called major energy circuit. The Chi thereby flows through the whole body from one meridian to the next, as in a closed system. Then the circulation starts anew.

As the Chi flows through the body continuously, the organs respond to external measures—such as acupuncture, Qigong, or Yin Yoga—at any time of day; but they do this best at their maximum times. For example, if you want to particularly strengthen the energy in the kidneys, then you should carry out your Yin Yoga practice for the kidneys and bladder meridian in the period from 3 to 7 p.m. (The bladder is the counterpart of the kidneys; the kidneys and bladder form a functional circuit and are assigned to the element of water—see page 29.)

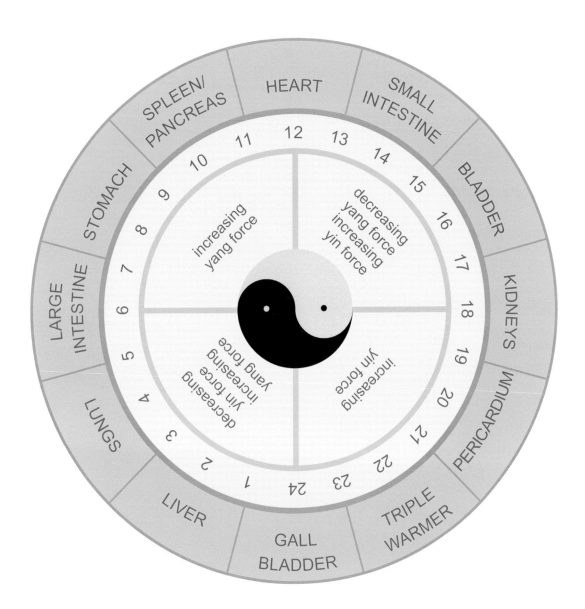

Each meridian has its own energetic peak phase. The organ clock can help you better categorize specific symptoms, or to find out the optimum time for targeted Yin Yoga practice or meridian massage (see page 36).

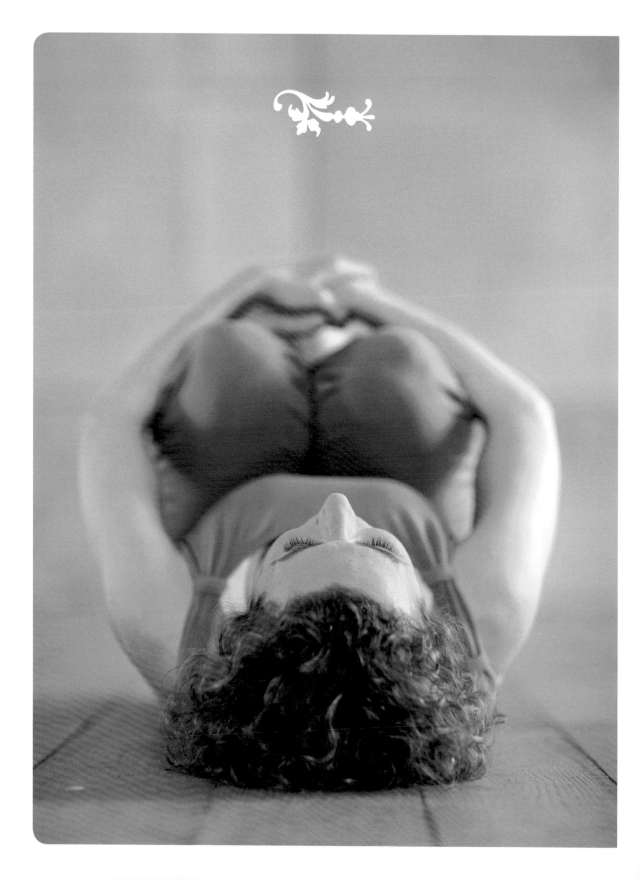

Yin Yoga
in Practice

In Yin Yoga, you can combine very different exercises and techniques with one another and adapt them to your individual needs at any time. Besides the classic Yin Yoga positions, I also present you here with some stimulating Yang positions that you can do now and then, as well as calming breathing techniques, gentle massages, and a small selection of meditations—everything you need for your healing and beneficial Yin Yoga practice.

❀ The **Massages**

Massages have a profound effect on our connective tissue, and they are also relaxing, releasing, and detoxifying. The following massage techniques offer you the opportunity to work directly on the meridians. And the best thing is that you do not need a partner or therapist for the massages, and only very little equipment. You can carry these out easily yourself—now and then, at any time, and daily if you wish.

❀ **Meridian Massage**

If symptoms become apparent at a specific meridian, it is advisable to pay particular attention to these. For example, if you keep suffering from a headache at the side of the head, then this pain would probably show up at the gallbladder meridian. As there are also always remote points for certain complaints, in this case you should include and massage the whole course of the meridian. Meridian massage can energize and harmonize the energy pathways and make them permeable. It moves the Chi and blood, and it can also have a positive effect on pain, release fascia that are stuck together, stimulate the metabolism and circulation, strengthen the immune system, move the lymph and vessel fluids, tone up the muscles, and strengthen the functions of the meridians.

Practicing the exercise

The meridians respond very well to pressing and kneading, but you can also handle them by pushing, rubbing, gripping, pinching, twisting, tapping, clapping, or stroking them, or combining different techniques with one another. Scraping is also possible, and this is best done with an aid such as a Gua Sha scraper, the lid of a marmalade jar, or a spoon. Do not worry: with this treatment, small bruises or considerable redness may arise. However, these are not usually painful and will disappear within a few days. In TCM, it is assumed that this has to do with waste products that are rising to the surface to be carried away. It is also possible you will feel tired after the meridian massage, in which case you should indulge yourself with a little rest. If you feel pain, then you have probably massaged too intensively or too long, so next time you should massage a little more gently and for a shorter period. If you have enough time it is very beneficial to work on the whole body, but you can also just stimulate individual meridians specifically.

If there is a lack of Chi, then the meridian should be worked on gently, cautiously, slowly, and for a longer time, in the direction of flow and in a clockwise direction—in this way you massage the Yin meridians from bottom to top, and the Yang meridians from top to bottom. Massaging in the direction of flow has a toning or stimulating effect on the Chi.

With a surplus of Chi, which you usually recognize by certain points on the course of the meridian being particularly painful, you do the opposite: stroke vigorously and quickly, against the flow of the meridian and in an anti-clockwise direction, to break down the abundance of Chi or draw it off so that a harmonious flow of energy can ensue. If you are unsure, then simply decide intuitively what feels better, or contact a TCM expert.

It is particularly effective to use the organ clock as a guide when doing the meridian massage (see page 36), and work on the meridians at the corresponding times. It is best to stimulate directly on the skin, perhaps with some body oil.

Before the massage, take a look at the precise course of the meridians that you wish to massage, and always massage both sides of the body. However, pay more attention to the side of the body on which you have the symptoms; the massage here may take a few minutes longer. The treatment should never cause a lot of pain, though! If that is the case, then please end the massage and contact a TCM expert to clarify the background.

Courses of the meridians

With meridian massage, you essentially work on the surface of the body, and you can therefore use the diagrams of the courses of the meridians on pages 30 and 31 to help you. However, as the meridians are all very close to one another and only a targeted massage ensures the best possible effect, I will describe the overall course of each individual meridian here.

The large intestine (**Yang**): the large intestine meridian begins on the outside of the nail of the index finger. It leads across the wrist to the outside of the forearm, to the point of the elbow, to the outside of the upper arm, to the shoulder and to the collarbone. It then goes to the level of the 7th cervical vertebrae and 1st thoracic vertebrae, and on to the spine. From there, the meridian leads back to the pit of the collarbone and runs deep down to the lungs, to the diaphragm, and to the large intestine. Another branch goes from the pit of the collarbone sideways to the throat, to the lower jaw, to the corner of the mouth, and down to the teeth of the lower jaw, and from the corner of the mouth to the upper lip and the wing of the nose, where it then passes to the stomach meridian.

Lungs **(Yin):** the lung meridian begins within the abdomen above the navel and runs down to the large intestine, up to the diaphragm and to the stomach. It flows on towards the lungs up to the throat and reaches the surface a thumb's width below the collarbone, near the shoulders in the upper body. From there it goes upwards a little and moves outwards over the front side of the shoulder above the bicep to the inside of the upper arm. It runs further across the crook of the arm and the inside of the forearm to the wrist, to the ball of the thumb, to the thumb, and ends at the inside of the tip of the thumb. Another branch goes from the wrist out to the outside of the index finger and runs from there into the large intestine meridian.

Stomach **(Yang):** the stomach meridian runs from the inside of the wing of the nose out to the inner corner of the eye and into the eye, comes out again and goes along the nose to the upper jaw, runs around the lips and goes to the lower jaw and jaw joint. One branch runs along from the ear at the level of the temple and into the forehead. Another branch runs through the body to the lungs, the diaphragm, the stomach, and the spleen. Another branch goes from the lower jaw to the chest, stomach, and groin. The branch that flows through the stomach joins together with another branch and runs from here down to the hips, the front side of the leg, and to the tip of the foot. The main branch goes to the outside of the second toe. Another branch flows to the inside of the big toe, where it passes into the spleen meridian.

Spleen **(Yin):** the spleen meridian begins at the inside of the big toe and flows across the bridge of the foot to the inside of the ankle, further up along the inside of the lower leg, to the inside of the knee and to the inside of the thigh, to the groin and stomach. One branch connects deeply with the spleen and stomach and runs to the diaphragm, collarbone, and armpit. Another branch runs deep into the collarbone, throat, and tongue. The next branch flows from the stomach out to the diaphragm and to the heart, where it connects with the heart meridian.

Small intestine **(Yang):** the small intestine meridian begins at the outside of the little finger and flows across the outside of the wrist to the forearm, the upper arm, the shoulder and shoulder blade, at the level of the 7th cervical vertebrae to the spine, and on to the collarbone. Here it goes deep into the heart, the trachea, the diaphragm, the stomach, and finally to the small intestine. One branch flows from the collarbone to the outside of the neck, to the cheek, to the outer corner of the eye, and to the ear. Another branch runs from the jaw to the cheek and on to the inner corner of the eye, where it connects with the bladder meridian.

Heart **(Yin):** the heart meridian begins at the heart and flows across the diaphragm to the small intestine. One branch runs from the heart to the throat and the eye. Another branch goes across the lungs to the armpit, and comes to the surface at the inside of the upper arm, goes to the crook of the arm, to the inside of the forearm, to the wrist, to the palm of the hand, and then to the inside of the little finger, where it connects with the small intestine meridian.

Bladder **(Yang):** the bladder meridian begins at the inner corner of the eye and flows across the forehead to the highest point of the skull. One branch goes from here to the brain, runs across the inside of the ear, through the back of the head to the neck, where it divides and runs down parallel to the spine (inner meridian). In the lower back, at the level of the lumbar spine, a branch runs inside and connects with the kidneys and bladder. Another branch goes from the lower back down to the buttocks, to the back of the thighs and the hollows of the knees, where it connects with another branch. From there it goes on to the rear side of the lower legs, to the outside of the ankles, to the outside of the feet, and to the outside of the little toes, where it connects with the kidney meridian. The branch that connects with the hollow of the knee flows next to the inner meridian from the neck and goes down to the spine (outer meridian), to the buttocks, to the hollows of the knees, to the back of the lower legs, to the outside of the ankles, to the outside of the feet, and then finally to the outside of the little toes, where it then connects with the kidney meridian.

Kidneys **(Yin):** the kidney meridian begins on the underside of the little toe and flows across the middle of the sole of the foot to the inside of the ankle, to the heel, the inside of the lower leg, the inside of the knee, the inside of the thigh, and up to the coccyx, where it connects inside with the kidneys and bladder. It leads on to the pubic bone, arrives at the surface of the stomach, and flows up to the liver, the diaphragm, chest, and collarbone. One branch goes from the kidneys to the liver, to the diaphragm, the lungs, the trachea, and the tongue. Another branch runs from the lungs to the heart and the pericardium, where it connects with the pericardium meridian.

Pericardium (Yin): the pericardium meridian begins in the heart and leads across the diaphragm to the lower abdomen. One branch runs from the heart across the chest, surfaces at the fourth rib, and leads to the armpit, to the inside of the upper arm, to the crook of the arm, to the inside of the forearm, to the palm of the hand, and to the tip of the middle finger. Another branch goes from the palm of the hand to the tip of the ring finger, where it connects with the triple warmer.

Triple warmer (Yang): this meridian is difficult for Westerners to grasp as it does not correspond to any organ. In TCM, the triple warmer is divided into an upper, middle, and lower warmer. It stands for absorption, processing, and excretion in the body and therefore has an effect on all important organs. The triple warmer begins at the outside of the ring finger and leads across the back of the hand to the wrist, to the outside of the forearm, to the elbow, to the outside of the upper arm, to the shoulder joint, to the shoulder and inside to the collarbone, to the pericardium, to the diaphragm, and on to the lower abdomen. One branch runs across the breastbone to the collarbone and to the neck, where it surfaces and goes to the throat and ear. On the inside it then runs to the hairline and the cheeks. Another branch goes from the ear into the inside of the ear, and runs from the ear to the outer corner of the eye, where it connects with the gallbladder meridian.

Gallbladder (Yang): the gallbladder meridian begins at the outer corner of the eye and runs to the ear and up to the hairline, across the side of the skull behind the ear, to the neck, the shoulder and then the collarbone. One branch runs behind the ear into the ear and back to the outer corner of the eye. From here another branch goes to the lower jaw, the cheek, the throat, the collarbone, the chest, the diaphragm, the liver, the gallbladder, the loins, the pubic bone, and finally to the hips. The next branch flows from the collarbone to the armpit, to the chest, the waist, the hip, the outside of the thigh, the outside of the knee, the outside of the lower leg, the outside of the ankle, and finally to the outside of the foot, up to the tip of the fourth toe. A small branch leads from the outside of the foot to the tip of the big toe, where it connects with the liver meridian.

Liver (Yin): the liver meridian begins at the outside of the big toe and flows across the bridge of the foot to the inside of the ankle, to the inside of the lower leg, to the inside of the knee, to the inside of the thigh, to the pubic bone, to the genitalia, to the lower abdomen, to the liver, and to the gallbladder. Inside it runs to the diaphragm, to the ribs, to the throat, to the pharynx, to the eyes, to the forehead, and finally to the top of the skull, where it connects with the governing vessel. One branch flows from the eyes across the nasal sinuses to the lips and goes around them. Another branch leads from the liver to the diaphragm and the lungs, where it connects with the lung meridian. Here the cycle begins again from the start.

Governing vessel (Yang): the governing vessel begins in the genital area. It surfaces at the perineal region and from there it runs to the back of the spine and to the head. One branch leads to the brain and on to the middle of the back of the head to the forehead, the nose, and the upper jaw.

Conception vessel (Yin): the conception vessel begins in the lower abdomen and comes to the surface in the perineal area. It flows across the pubic bone to the stomach, the throat, the lower jaw, and goes around the mouth, and from here it runs to the cheek and eye.

Meridian Tapping Massage

Meridian tapping massage is another technique for activating the flow of energy, in which you tap at or smooth out the meridians repeatedly with the hands or fingers along the course of the energy pathways. It is a very stimulating exercise.

Practicing the exercise

Stand comfortably and stretch one arm straight out in front of you. Tap the inside of the arm a few times from the shoulder down to the hand, and the outside from the hand back up to the shoulder. Then change sides.

Then tap on your breastbone using your fingers. It is said that tapping the breastbone every day activates the thymus gland that is located behind it and therefore strengthens the immune system. Then include the other hand and tap on your whole chest. If you wish, you can also make a sound while doing this on a long exhalation. Open your mouth and let out a sound intuitively. Then bring your hands to your stomach and start tapping or smoothing the ribcage gently from the lower right upwards (ascending large intestine), then straight to the left underneath the ribs (transverse large intestine) and then back down again (descending large intestine). Now take the hands to your back and tap your kidneys or smooth your hands over them.

Open your legs a little wider and bend forward. Now tap the inside of the legs a few times from the ankles upwards, and on the outside from the buttocks back down to the ankles. Then tap the front side of

> #### ∽ **Important!** ∽
>
> In the following cases, you should not carry out a meridian massage or meridian tapping massage, or you should discuss it with a TCM doctor or therapist to clarify your individual situation.
>
> - During pregnancy (do not do the massage during the first three months, and after the first three months avoid the lumbar spine and sacral region)
> - If you suffer from osteoporosis (gentle massage only)
> - With infectious skin diseases and infectious illnesses
> - If you have open wounds or burns
> - In the event of fever
> - In cases of extreme tension or nervousness
> - With heart conditions
> - With illnesses that are associated with an increased tendency to bleed or with severe circulatory conditions

the legs from ankles up to the groin, and on the rear of the legs from the buttocks back down to the ankles. Stand straight again and bend one leg, cross the other one over it, and now tap on the bridge of the foot and the sole of the foot. If you find it difficult to balance, you can sit on the floor for this massage.

Then bring the fingertips to your head and tap from the forehead across the skull to the neck. Then use your fingers to tap your whole face very gently—this is very beneficial, particularly under the eyes and on the jaw joints.

Now lower your hands and feel into it; sense the energy in your hands. Then bend the arms and bring the palms of the hands closer together. Feel the energy field between your hands, which may feel something like a ball of energy. Play with this ball: take the hands closer together again and then apart, and see how far you can feel this energy field. Then bring the palms of the hands close together to compress the energy. Now bring this compressed energy to a place on your body where you know it is required—for example, where you experience pain or blockages. If nothing occurs to you, or if you feel quite healthy, you can take your hands to the center of energy in your abdomen. Lay your hands flat on it and let the energy radiate in.

Stomach Massage

An alternative to the meridian massage is the stomach massage. You can use this to stimulate your stomach organs and the meridians running through the abdomen; it encourages digestion in particular, and helps with detoxification. You can work directly with your hands, or use a ball. Carry out the stomach massage daily if you like, but do not do it during pregnancy. With stomach massage it is important to listen to your body well—you will then easily discover how much pressure is right to use, and how intensive or gentle the movements should be.

Practicing the exercise

For the **stomach massage**, lie back comfortably on the floor **with your hands** at your side and relax your stomach. Then place your hands on your abdomen and let them rest there for a moment with the initial contact. Let the breath flow into your hands. Now start to massage. Proceed in a clockwise direction, as that is the natural course for the digestion. Start from the lower right at the ascending large intestine, then go upwards to the ribcage, massage the transverse large intestine in a straight line, and then move to the left side to the descending large intestine, moving downwards. You then start from the beginning again. You can use your flat hands or fingertips to do this. Use oil, if you wish. Your abdomen also likes circling movements, or the type of massage known as "rolling folds of skin." To do this, take a fold of skin between your fingertips and roll it to and fro in different directions. This makes the skin more elastic. Before and after massaging, you should always drink at least one glass of water to flush out toxins well.

    To do the **stomach massage using a ball**, you will require a soft ball—for example, a Pilates ball. Lie with your stomach on the ball. It is important to completely relax and allow deep breathing to take place to withstand the resistance of the ball. After every fifth to eighth breath, move the ball so that, bit by bit, you massage the whole abdomen. This exercise stimulates the flow of lymph and therefore the entire immune system. This also has a strong detoxifying effect and regulates the entire digestive system. In addition, you can use this technique very effectively to soften scar tissue in the stomach area and discourage growths. The massage is also effective at a mental level; it can bring buried emotions back to the surface. To judge by recent findings, diabetics also benefit from it: you can greatly lower the blood sugar level—I have been able to observe this for myself with a diabetic, who measured her values before and after rolling.

❋ The **Yin Yoga Positions**

The Yin positions have a balancing effect; they stimulate the meridians and harmonize the flow of energy. The meridians mentioned may always vary a little, depending on how a position is implemented. Do the following exercises without any pressure to perform at all, and allow yourself to be led by your inner yoga teacher. When practicing, you can either work with the suggested sequences or just select a few exercises. The holding time of the poses is just a suggestion; if you want, you can vary it, of course.

❦ Ankle Stretch and Toe Stretch (Vajrasana)

The heel and toe stretches intensively extend the toes and the plantar fascia, the fascia in the soles of the feet. They strengthen the ankles and are also a good remedy for cold feet. If the position causes you major difficulties, then I recommend doing it more often for a certain period, maybe even daily—often we only find it difficult as we are no longer used to this sitting position.

Effect

The position addresses the individual meridians in the toes and the soles of the feet—the spleen, liver, stomach, gallbladder, bladder, and kidney meridians.

Practicing the exercise

1. Sit on your heels; if you are sensitive here, you can also place a blanket underneath. Straighten your upper body and let your weight fall onto your feet with your hands resting on your legs. If you find the **Ankle Stretch** too intense, shift forward a bit more and place your hands on the floor. If you want to feel more of a stretch, then take the hands behind your feet and raise the knees.

2. Then come into the opposite position and place the balls of the feet so that the toes are directed upwards. If the little toe is in the air then pull it forward gently with the fingers. Take the hands in front of the knee if the pressure is too strong in the **Toe Stretch**.

3 and 4. Feel free to try out the positions in both versions that **stretch your fingers, arms, and shoulders:** stretch one arm out long and extend the individual fingers on both hands. Then grip your hands behind your back; alternatively you can do this using a belt.

5. Then lean forward with a straight back and place the backs of your hands on the floor so that the fingers are about in line with your knees. You can then **stretch the wrists**.

6. If you have pain in the knees with this exercise then either sit higher—on two **blocks** or on a **yoga bolster**, for example, which you place between the thigh and lower leg.

Remain in the heel and toe stretch for two to four minutes (less if it is too intense), including the versions with the finger, arm, shoulder, and wrist stretch. Finally, loosen your ankles by circling them in both directions several times. Then keep your hands and feet still and relax for a few breaths.

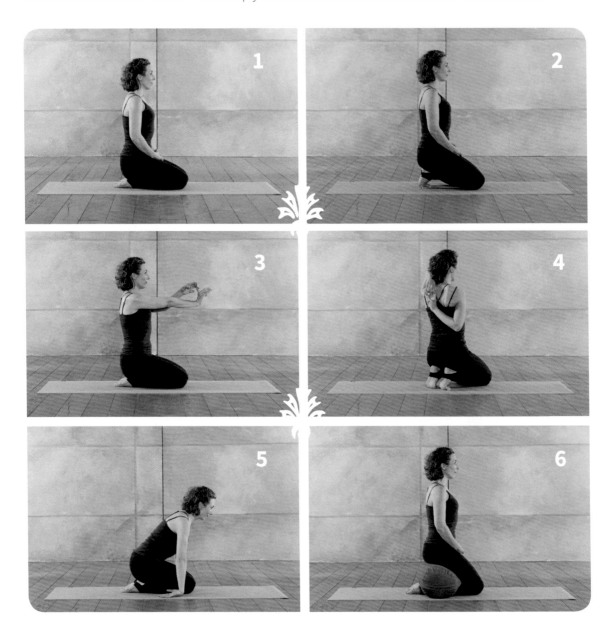

❀ **Bridge** (Setu Bandha Sarvangasana)

This position opens up the thoracic spine, the heart chamber, and the shoulders.

Effect

The stretch is particularly effective for the meridians of the stomach, spleen, kidneys, liver, lungs, heart, and pericardium.

Practicing the exercise

Place a yoga bolster lengthways on the mat and a block at the lower end of the mat. Sit at the lower end of the yoga bolster and lean back so that your shoulder blades are on the upper end of the bolster. Place your shoulders and head on the floor. Rest your head on a blanket or small cushion if the position is uncomfortable for the cervical spine. Take your arms back above you slowly and place them next to your head.

Stay in Bridge for three to five minutes. Either push yourself up gently with an activated pelvic floor, or roll out of the position sideways. Place the props to one side and come into Relaxed Supine Position (see page 87), relaxing into it.

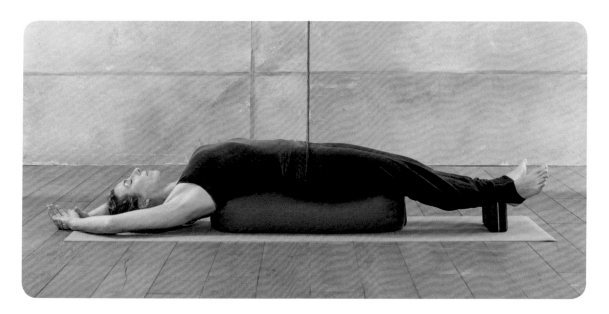

❦ **Butterfly** (Baddha Konasana)

The position stretches the entire back and the insides of the legs. It is particularly good for women during menstruation, and is also a suitable yoga position in pregnancy.

Effect

Butterfly works on the meridians of the liver, kidneys, spleen, and bladder. The side bend and rotation also stimulate the gallbladder meridian and, in the sidebend, the small intestine, large intestine, and triple warmer meridian.

Practicing the exercise

1. Sit on the mat, place the soles of your feet together, and pull the feet towards the pelvis. Let the knees drop gently outwards, or support the outsides of the legs with two blocks if this stretch is too intense for you. You can also sit on a blanket or a cushion. Relax the back, let your upper body sink forward passively, and place your arms where it is comfortable for you.

2. If you want to try more variations, straighten up again and come into a **side bend**. Place the left hand next to the left knee and lean leftwards with your upper body. Leave the right arm behind your back or take it above the head for more stretch. Then change sides and perform the side bend to the right.

3. You can also combine Butterfly with an active **rotation**. To do this, grip your right knee with your left hand, place your right hand behind the pelvis, and turn rightwards with a straight spine. Then change sides and carry out the rotation to the left.

4. In addition to the stretch, you can also activate the bubbling spring **acupressure point** with your fingers; this is the kidney point on the sole of the foot, which is located centrally directly underneath the ball of the foot. It counteracts anxiety and exhaustion, clears and calms the mind, and has a grounding effect.

Remain in Butterfly for three to five minutes, including the rotation and the side bend. Alternatively, you can also stay in the forward bend only. Press the acupressure point gently as long as it feels good. Then come back to the center and extend both legs again. Relax into Supine Position (see page 87).

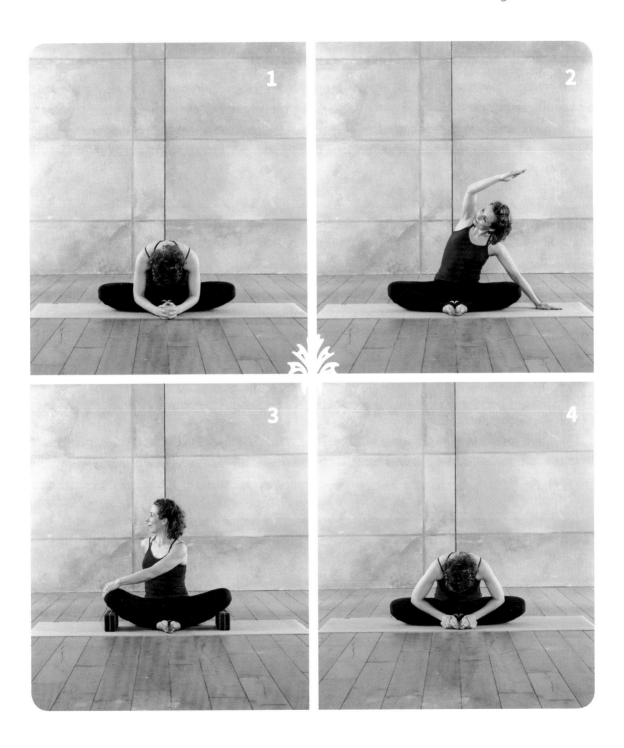

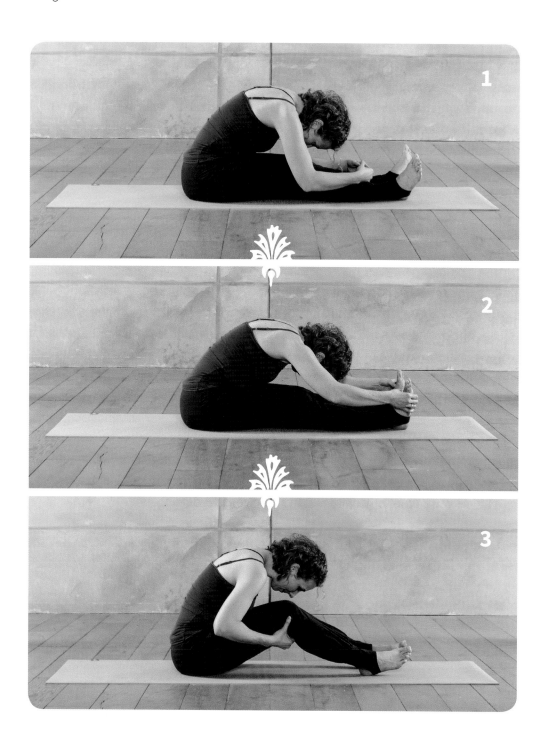

❀ Chair exercises

These gentle versions of the classic exercises are excellent for people with reduced mobility or for older people.

Practicing the exercise

1. Gentle Dangling Pose: Sit on the front edge of the chair, bend the knees, and place the feet hip width apart firmly on the floor. Support your forearms on your thighs and bend forward with a rounded spine. Relax the shoulders and neck area. Roll yourself up again and relax.

2. Long Dangling Pose: Long dangling pose is more intense than the gentle version. Stay seated on the front edge of the chair and stretch your legs out long. Bend forward again, and either let your forearms lie on your thigh or take the upper body between the legs and your hands to the floor. Roll up again slowly and relax.

3. Side bend: Sit sideways on the chair so that you can place your right arm on the back of the chair. Your feet should be hip width apart and the knees bent. Now tilt your upper body to the right and take the left arm long above the head. Leave your head relaxed so that you can also stretch the side of the neck at the same time. Then change sides. Come back to the center and relax.

4. Backbend: Stand behind the chair so that you can grip the chair with your hands. Now move back step by step until your back forms a straight line. If this feels difficult, then bend the knees until you can notice a stretch in the back and shoulders. Let your breath become deep and calm. Come back towards the chair, straighten up, and circle your shoulders in both directions a few times.

5. Rotation: Sit on the front edge of the chair so that your feet are placed firmly on the floor. Straighten your spine and turn towards the right while gripping the chair with your right hand. The right shoulder is pulled back, the left one is forward, and your crown is directed upwards. Let the breath flow deeply and calmly. Change sides and then relax.

6 and 7. Hip-opener (inner): Sit on the chair and open your legs out as wide as possible. Bend your upper body forward between your legs, keeping your back rounded. If necessary, place some props in front of the chair to give height. Relax the shoulder and neck area and let your head go forward loosely. Roll out again and relax.

8. Hip-opener (outer): Sit on the front of the chair, bend your left knee, and place your foot firmly on the floor. Now place your right leg angled on the left thigh, with the right knee pointing outwards. Bend forward with a rounded back and place the arms on your legs. Relax the shoulder and neck area. Then change sides. Roll out again and relax.

9. Relaxed supine position: Lie on your back, bring your buttocks close to the chair, bend your knees, and place the lower leg on the seat. Take your hands onto your stomach, or place them stretched out long next to the body. Give your weight completely to the floor and relax. Alternatively, you can also assume the position lying on the bed or on a couch, and place a yoga bolster under the backs of your knees.

Remain in the position as long as it feels good.

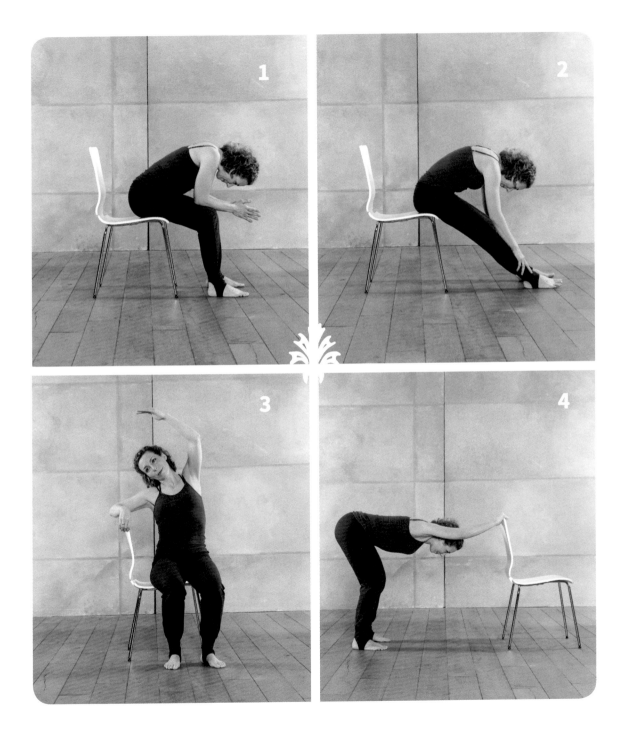

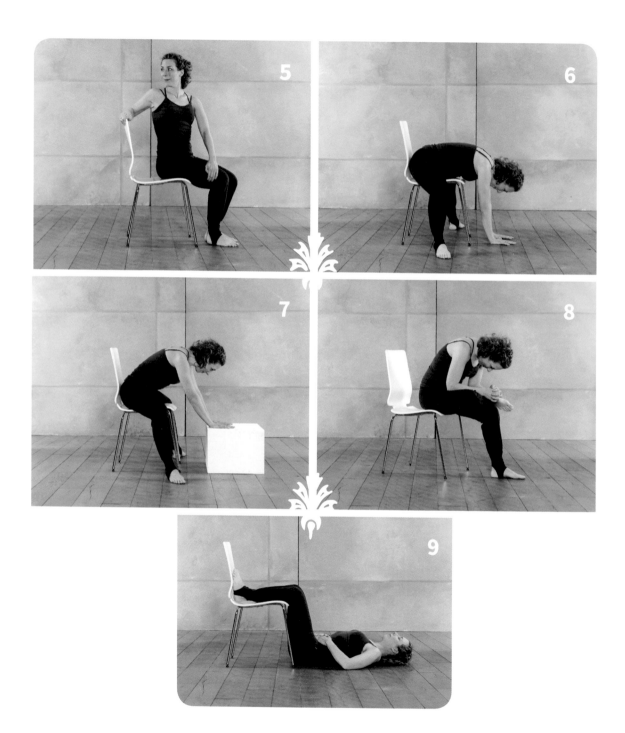

❋ Child's Pose (Balasana)

Child's Pose is good if you need time to recover or if you wish to neutralize between exercises. The position relaxes the back, shoulders, and neck. It stretches the bridges of the foot and the ankles, relaxes the spine, and evenly massages the stomach organs.

Effect

In Child's Pose, the focus is on the bladder meridian.

Practicing the exercise

In the classic Child's Pose, sit on your heels and let your upper body sink forward. Your arms are stretched out relaxed next to your legs, and your forehead touches the floor. If you wish, you can put a blanket underneath you. Alternatively, you can place one fist on top of the other and place your forehead on them. Keep your legs closed or open, whichever feels more comfortable.

In a gentle version that is also suitable in pregnancy or during menstruation, you use a yoga bolster or a rolled-up blanket. You take the bolster between your legs and place your upper body on top of it. You can now support your head on your hands or taper the bolster a little by placing a yoga block under it. Alternatively, cross your arms under the bolster and place your head on it, facing sideways. Then change sides in between, so that the cervical spine can also rotate in the other direction.

Remain in the position as long as it feels good and then roll out of it again slowly.

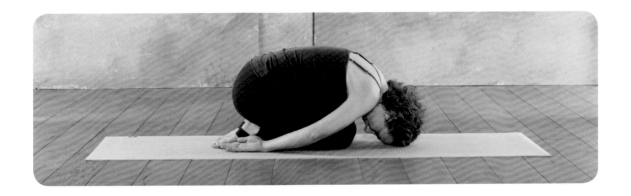

❁ **Crane** (Ardha Malasana)

This exercise opens up the pelvic area and stretches the groin as well as the inside of the legs. It also massages and stimulates the stomach organs.

Effect

Crane works on the meridians of the liver, kidneys, spleen, and bladder in particular. With the rotation and the side bend the gallbladder meridian is stimulated too, and the side bend with the lifted arm also has an effect on the small intestine meridian, the large intestine meridian, and the triple warmer.

Practicing the exercise

1. Come into the basic position: your left leg is bent as in the squat, and the right leg is stretched out to the side or slightly bent at the knee. To make the position easier, you can also sit on a yoga bolster or a rolled-up blanket. Then bend forward with a relaxed upper body.

2. If you want to do other variations, then come into a **side bend**, where you are sitting up straight again, and take your right arm to your right leg. Now tilt your upper body right and take the left arm above your head or behind your back.

3. Sit up straight again to carry out Crane with a **rotation**. Grip your right leg or the yoga bolster with your left hand, and place your right hand behind the pelvis with your arm stretched. Your spine should remain straight.

Stay in Crane for three to five minutes, including the side bend and the stretch. Then turn back to the center and repeat the process on the other side. Alternatively, you can simply remain in the front bend. To conclude, relax into Supine Position (see page 87).

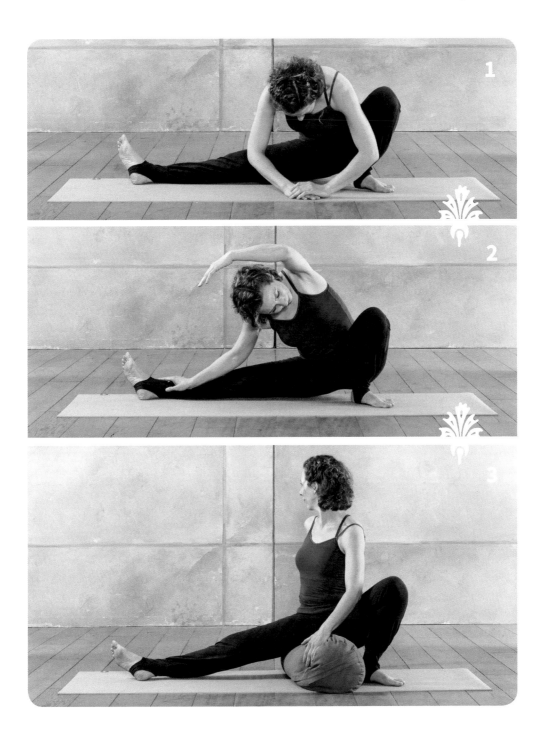

❦ **Dangling** (Uttanasana)

This exercise stretches the whole rear side of the body and gently presses the stomach organs together at the same time, which has a massaging effect and supports the digestion. As with Caterpillar (see page 51), it works on all the long fascia chains on the rear side of the body, and the hanging also releases the neck nicely.

Effect

Dangling, also known as standing forward bend, intensively stimulates the bladder meridian and also works on the small intestine, the large intestine, and the triple warmer meridian, provided you include the arms.

Practicing the exercise

1. Stand upright, open the legs to hip width, relax the back, and bend your upper body downwards to the thighs. Do not tighten up, but simply let yourself sink down gently. If the stretch is too strong on the backs of your thighs, you can bend the knees slightly. Let your arms either hang down long or cross them loosely. Keep your head and neck completely relaxed in the position. For a gentler version, you can also put a yoga bolster between your body and legs.

2. Alternatively, you can also combine Dangling with an **arm stretch**. Grip your hands behind your back and let your outstretched arms drop forward towards your head.

Remain in the position for three to five minutes. Then bend the legs and roll your upper body up slowly. Come into a neutral position and relax into Supine Position (see page 87).

> ❦ **Important:** please refrain from this position if you have increased intraocular pressure. You should also take particular care if you suffer from high blood pressure. If your blood pressure is too low, you should not roll up to release; it is better to sit down. In both cases, if you feel uncomfortable in this position, Caterpillar (see page 51) is a good alternative. ❦

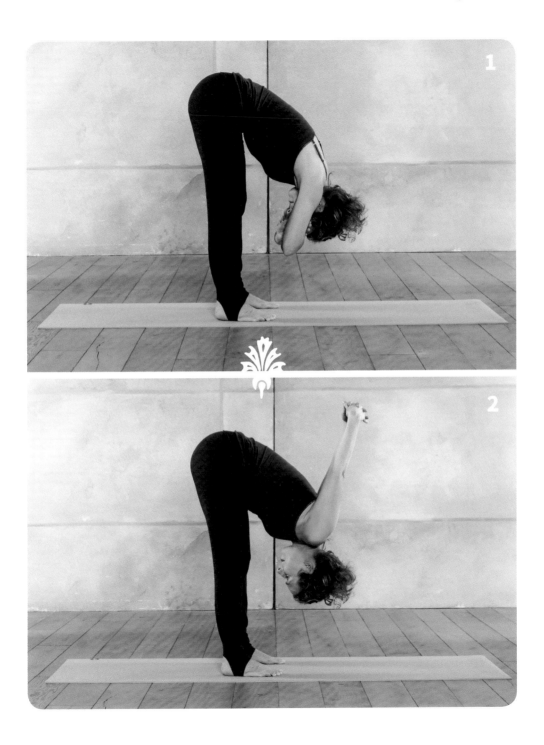

✻ **Dragon** (Anjaneyasana)

Dragon is one of the more intense positions, as the Yang element can clearly be felt here. This is absolutely okay, as there is always some Yang in all Yin, and vice versa. But try to reduce the Yang element as much as you can by allowing yourself to go into the pose in the best way possible, or by using props.

Effect

With Dragon, the focus is on the meridians of the stomach, spleen, liver, kidneys, gallbladder, and bladder, depending on the version you practice. It intensively stretches the groin, the fronts of the thighs, and the bridge of the feet, and (depending on the variation) the upper body, buttocks, and hip area as well. Dragon is also a very good preparation for Saddle (see page 90).

Practicing the exercise

1 and 2. Come onto all fours, and place a blanket under the knees if you are sensitive to pressure here. Then take your right leg from between your hands and place your left knee on the floor. If you want the position to be gentler, then pull the left knee forward slightly; for more intensity, take it further back. The right knee can be placed in front of, above, or behind the ankle, but this should not cause any pain in the knee. Let the pelvis sink towards the floor very passively. Now place the hands either left or right next to the foot, or both on the inside. The position becomes more intense if you support yourself on your forearms, and it is slightly easier if you use props—for example, **blocks** or a **yoga bolster**.

3. If you want to intensify **the backbend**, you can put your hands on the front of your thigh for support.

4. For the version that includes a **rotation**, place your right hand on the right knee and turn your upper body to the right while looking upwards.

As Dragon is a rather intense exercise, I recommend trying different variations. Remain on the right side for three to five minutes, including the backbend and rotation versions, and then repeat the sequence with the left leg forward. To release or to change sides, you can either go into Downward

Facing Dog (see page 115) or into Child's Pose (see page 57). Then move slowly into Resting Forward Pose (see page 88).

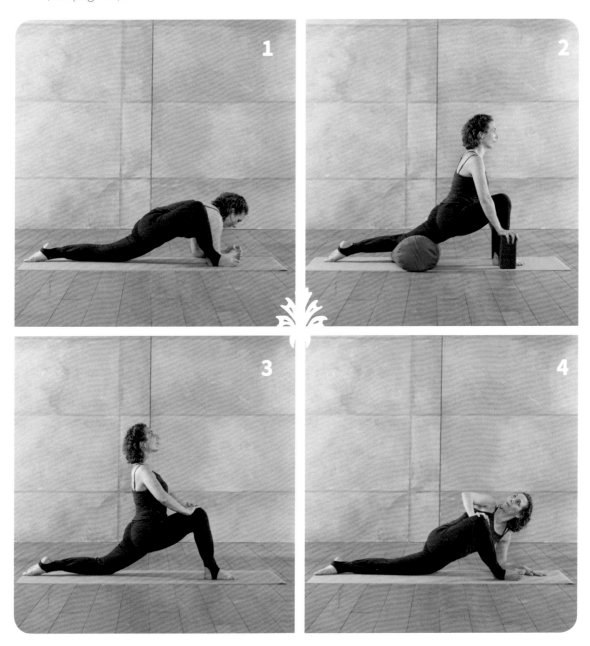

✤ **Dragonfly** (Upavistha Konasana)

This position is very beneficial for women during menstruation, as it opens the pelvic area wide and relaxes it. This provides a harmonizing effect for abdominal or hormone-related complaints, for men as well as women. By using props you can also massage the stomach and abdominal organs.

Effect

Dragonfly mainly works on the meridians of the liver, kidneys, spleen, and bladder. With the rotation and side bend, the gallbladder is also stimulated, and the side bend with the lifted arm has an effect on the small intestine meridian, the large intestine meridian, and the triple warmer.

Practicing the exercise

1. Sit on the mat with outstretched legs, and open your legs wide until you feel a comfortable stretch in the sides of the legs. Take a yoga bolster or a rolled-up blanket and lay it centrally lengthways in front of you so that your stomach is touching the bolster when you bend forward. If you want to massage the lower stomach organs, then lay the bolster flat on the floor. You can reach the upper stomach organs better if you place one or two blocks under the lower end of the bolster. If you are not very mobile, you can also place additional blankets or blocks on the bolster to raise it. Then relax your back and legs, and bend forward as far as your body will allow. Rest your head on your hands or props. Direct your breath gently to the stomach and pelvic area.

2. Alternatively, you can also go into **Half Dragonfly** by stretching your leg out to the side and bending the other one inwards, pulling your foot to your pelvis. You can then also change the position of the leg.

3. Another variation is Dragonfly with a **side bend**. Sit up straight again and tilt your upper body to the left. Place the bolster on the left leg so that your arm is supported comfortably. You can either take your right arm behind your back, or lift it at an angle over the head to increase the stretch.

4. Sit up straight again and stretch the spine to combine Dragonfly with a **rotation**. Place your left hand in front of or on your right leg, and your right hand behind the pelvis. You then look over your shoulder.

5. If the position feels difficult, then you can also go into a supine position. Sit on a yoga bolster or by a wall. Lie backwards onto your back, and raise the legs upwards or bring them to the wall. Now open your legs and let gravity do the rest of the work.

Remain in Dragonfly for three to five minutes, including Dragonfly in the supine position or Half Dragonfly, and changing sides. You can stay in the side bend for one to two minutes per side, and in the rotation for around five to eight breaths. Then come back to the center and relax into Supine Position (see page 87). Alternatively, you can just do the forward bend.

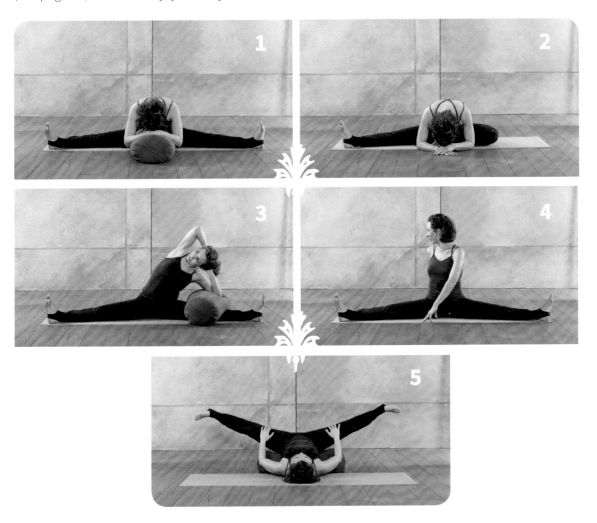

❀ Easy Pose with arm and shoulder stretch (Sukhasana)

This position opens up the hips and stretches the whole back as well as the arms and shoulders.

Effect

Easy Pose with arm and shoulder stretch works on the meridians of the gallbladder, bladder, lungs, heart, pericardium, small intestine, large intestine, and the triple warmer.

Practicing the exercise

1. Come into Easy Pose, your right arm crossed in front of the left. To make the position more comfortable, you can also place a cushion under the buttocks and support your knees by raising them. Bend forward in a relaxed way with a rounded back, and cross your arms so that your right arm is in front of your left arm and the palms are facing upwards. Alternatively, you can grip the opposite shoulder.

2. Then change the arm position by placing the palms downwards on the opposite knees.

Remain in Easy Pose for three to five minutes, including both arm positions. Then straighten up again, release the arms and legs, and move to and fro loosely a few times. Then change sides—crossing the left leg in front of the right one, and the left arm in from of the right—and repeat the process.

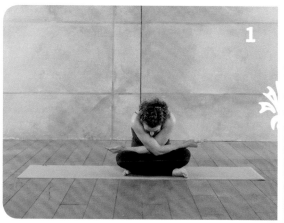
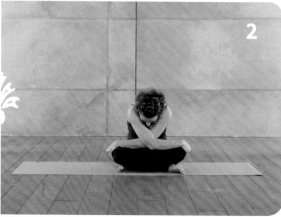

❋ Embracing Wings

This position stretches the arms and shoulders. It is one of the few Yin Yoga exercises that reaches the outsides of the arms and therefore the meridians that run through there.

Effect

Embracing Wings has a particular effect on the meridians of the small intestine, large intestine, and triple warmer.

Practicing the exercise

Lie on your stomach and cross your outstretched arms at shoulder height under your body. Your right arm is in front of the left one, and your palms are facing upwards. Place a block or folded blanket under your forehead, or a yoga bolster under your chest if you wish. Give your weight up to the floor. If the tips of your fingers go numb in this position, then you should change it—for example, with the head up higher or moving your arms a few centimeters up or down.

Remain in the position for two to three minutes and then change sides. Release your arms again and then relax into Supine Position (see page 87).

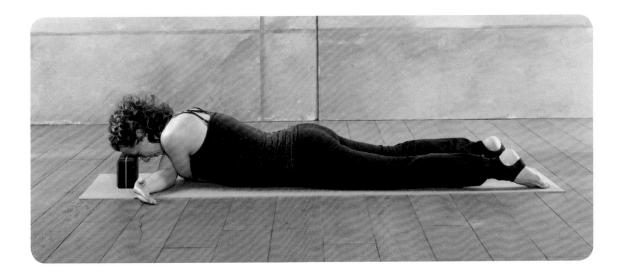

❀ **Eye of the Needle** (Sucirandharasana)

This position mobilizes the hip joints and gently massages the abdomen. The version that includes the outstretched leg also stretches the back of the leg, and the stomach organs are stimulated when it is combined with a rotation.

Effect

With Eye of the Needle, the focus is on the meridians of the gallbladder and bladder, and possibly also on the liver, kidneys, and spleen. With the arms, the lungs, heart, and pericardium are also stimulated.

Practicing the exercise

1. Sit on a yoga bolster or a rolled-up blanket, and take your upper body back onto the floor. Your arms are stretched out long next to your head. Lift your feet from the floor and cross the right leg over the left, then let your knee sink down to your chest. You can hold the position effortlessly by elevating the pelvis slightly.

2. Alternatively you can stretch your left leg out long, if the position is more comfortable for you that way.

3. Place the bolster to the side to combine Eye of the Needle with a **rotation**. Hold the legs in the crossed position and then let the left knee drop and sink down to the left side. Turn your head to the right if you wish to feel more of a stretch; your arms remain relaxed on the floor. Let your breath become calm and even.

Stay in the position for three to five minutes, including the rotated version. Loosen the legs from one another and then change sides. Finally, relax into Supine Position (see page 87).

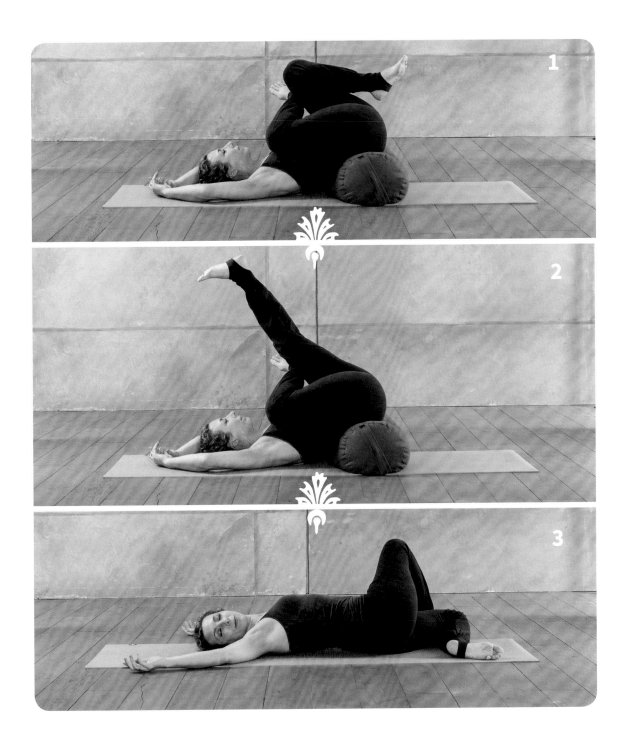

❀ **Fish** (Matsyasana)

With this exercise, you stretch the front side of your upper body, thereby supporting the flow of the breath and organ functions.

Effect

Fish has an effect on the meridians of the stomach, spleen, kidneys, liver, lungs, heart, and pericardium.

Practicing the exercise

Place a yoga bolster or a rolled-up blanket straight across the mat, and place a block at the head end. Sit in front of the bolster, lean backwards, and position yourself in such a way that your shoulder blades are comfortably on the bolster. Lay your head on the block and take your arms slowly behind or next to your head.

Stay in the position for three to five minutes. To come out of it, take the arms back to your body, and either come back up with an activated pelvic floor or roll out of the position sideways. Place the props to the side and then feel your way into Relaxed Supine Position (see page 87).

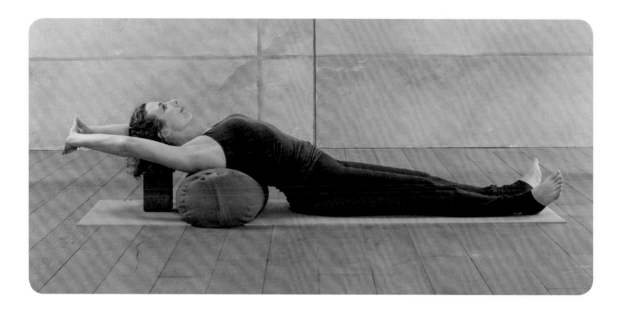

✤ **Frog** (Bhekasana)

This position opens up the pelvic area, and can therefore have a harmonizing effect on the organs in the abdomen.

Effect

Frog has an effect on the meridians of the liver, kidneys, spleen, and bladder.

Practicing the exercise

1. Place a yoga bolster or thickly rolled blanket lengthways on the mat. Sit on the bolster, the heels under the buttocks or a little further to the sides, with the knees opened as widely as possible so that it is comfortable. Take the buttocks to the front end of the bolster, and bend your rounded upper body forward so that you can support yourself with the arms. Feel the gentle stretch on the sides of the legs. For a more intense stretch, you can also go into this position directly on the floor without a bolster.

2. You can also do Frog with a **rotation**. To do this, take the left arm through the right and place your left shoulder on the floor until you feel an extension of the spine. Then change sides and turn to the left.

Stay in this position for three to five minutes, including the rotated version to the right and left. Bring one knee after the other back to the center, and come into Relaxed Supine Position (see page 87) or into Resting Forward Pose (see page 88) to relax into it.

(Pose shown on next page)

Frog *(described on page 71)*

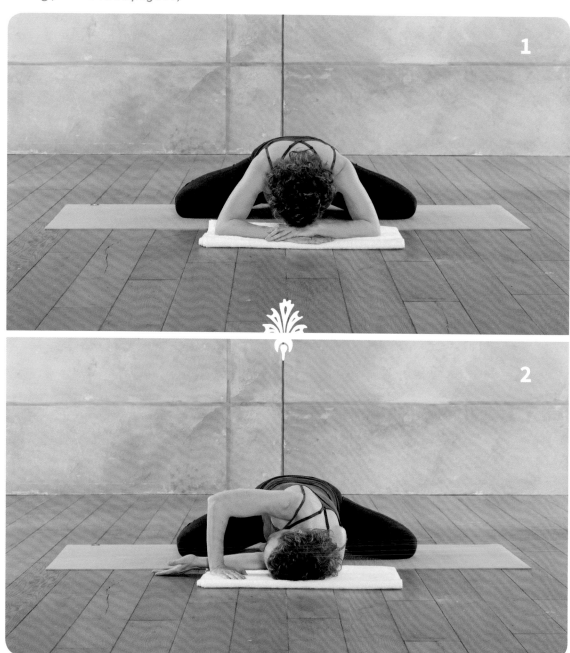

✤ **Half Butterfly** (Janu Shirshasana)

The position stimulates the kidneys, liver, and spleen, as well as the ascending and descending large intestine. It also stretches the insides and backs of the legs.

Effect

Half Butterfly has an effect on the meridians of the bladder, liver, and kidneys. With the rotation and side bend, the gallbladder is also stimulated. The side bend also activates the small intestine meridian, the large intestine meridian, and the triple warmer.

Practicing the exercise

1. Sit on the mat with legs outstretched, and slightly raised on a blanket or cushion if you wish. Bend your right leg so that the heel is pointing towards the center of your pelvis. Place a block or the yoga bolster under the bent leg if there is too much tension there. Then relax your back and allow yourself to sink forward passively towards your outstretched leg.

2. Alternatively you can also bend your right leg outwards in Half Butterfly, if this makes the position more comfortable for you.

3. If you want to try other variations, then sit upright again and go into a **side bend**. While doing this, maintain the position of the legs, turn your upper body towards the bent right leg, and then tilt it towards the outstretched left leg. You can prop yourself up with your bent left arm on the left leg or on a cushion; the right arm is outstretched above the head to the left side or remains behind your back.

4. Then come into an active **rotation**. Sit up straight again and grip the outside of your bent right leg (at around knee height) with your left hand. Place your right hand behind your pelvis and stabilize yourself in this position.

Remain in the position for three to five minutes, including the side bend and the rotation. Come back to the center, stretch your leg out again, and move to and fro a few times. Then change sides and carry out both versions of the exercise. Alternatively you can also remain in the front bend only. Then relax into Supine Position (see page 87). *(Pose shown on next page)*

Half Butterfly *(described on page 73)*

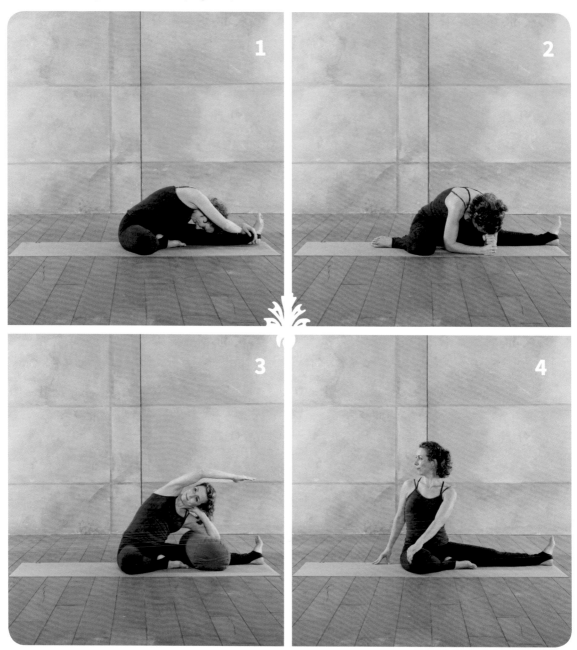

❋ Half Lying Lotus (Supta Ardha Padmasana)

Half Lying Lotus opens your pelvis area and has a relaxing effect, supplying the abdominal organs with blood. You also stretch your chest area in this position, which can help you breathe deeply.

Effect

The focus here is on the meridians of the gallbladder, stomach, spleen, liver, kidneys, lungs, heart, and pericardium.

Practicing the exercise

Place your yoga bolster or a rolled-up blanket lengthways on the mat, and sit in front of it with a small gap behind. Sit cross-legged and place your right foot on the inside of the left thigh. If you find this stretch too intense, you can place the foot on your lower leg or remain in the classic cross-legged position. Lie back in the raised position and place something underneath your head. Take the arms back slowly next to your head or to the side, so that you feel a stretch in the chest and shoulder area. If your fingertips feel numb, take your arms back to your sides or place them on your stomach.

Remain in the position for three to five minutes. Take your arms back to your sides, push yourself upwards with an activated pelvic floor, and bend your upper body forward for a few breaths to balance out. Sit upright, stretch your legs out, and move back and forth a few times. Then cross your legs the other way around and repeat the exercise.

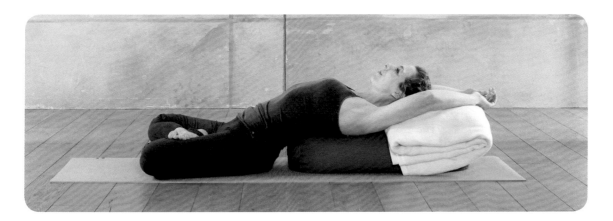

❧ **Happy Baby** (Ananda Balasana)

This position opens the pelvis area and mobilizes the hip joints. The liver, spleen, and ascending as well as descending large intestine are gently massaged, and the lower back is stretched. Not everyone can grip their feet as shown in the image. However, this is not necessary, as there should only be stimulation from the stretch on the outside of the legs; for some of those practicing it, there will be stimulation on the inside of the legs, too. The feelings may turn out to be very different with this exercise, depending on the position assumed. That is absolutely fine as there is no right or wrong, and the meridians are reached in any case.

Effect

Happy Baby is particularly effective for the meridians of the gallbladder and bladder, and possibly also for the liver, kidneys, and spleen. Rocking gently to and fro in the position can also have a very relaxing effect and calm the mind.

Practicing the exercise

1. Lie on the mat in the back position, and bend your legs so that the knees are on either side of your upper body. If the hip joints do not allow that, then simply open the legs as wide as you possibly can. Take the hands to the soles of your feet, which are now facing the ceiling, or use a yoga belt, and pull downwards gently. You can draw the feet a little more towards your head, if you want to feel the stretch in your lower back. If this is not possible, then grip the back of your thighs instead. If the stretch is too intense for you, then bring the soles of the feet together to change the opening of the pelvic area. Either stay still in the position or rock gently back and forth; you can also stretch each leg while the other remains bent.

2. Alternatively, you can try **Half Happy Baby**. In this position you only bend one leg while the other remains stretched out on the floor; you can also take a yoga belt to hold the foot. Then change sides. The exercise is more accessible this way for some, while it can also be more intensive for others.

Hold the position for three to five minutes, and for Half Happy Baby, three to five minutes on each side. Then release the hands from the feet, stretch the legs out again, and relax into Supine Position (see page 87).

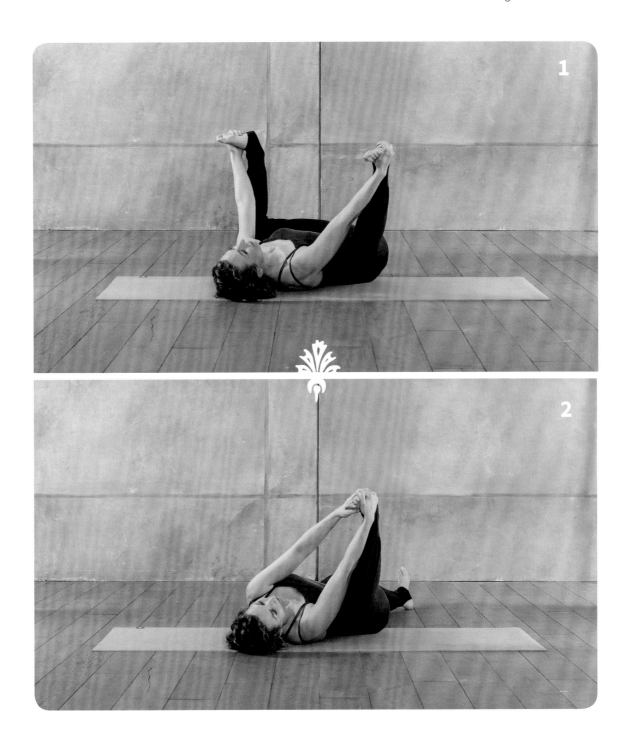

Lying Banana (Bananasana)

In this position the side stomach organs—the liver and spleen, the ascending and descending large intestine, and the lobe of the lung—are stretched on one side, and compressed on the other side.

Effect

Lying Banana works on the meridians of the gallbladder, small intestine, large intestine, and triple warmer.

Practicing the exercise

Place a yoga bolster or a rolled-up blanket straight across your mat and sit to the right of the bolster. Now tilt your upper body left and place yourself in a relaxed way on the bolster. Your head rests on your left arm, which you can also support with a blanket. Bend your legs comfortably, or (for more opening of the hips) take them to a 90-degree angle. Stretch out your right arm leftwards over your head. Let your weight go downwards.

Hold the position for three to five minutes, then push yourself back up and change sides. Place your props to one side and relax into Supine Position (see page 87).

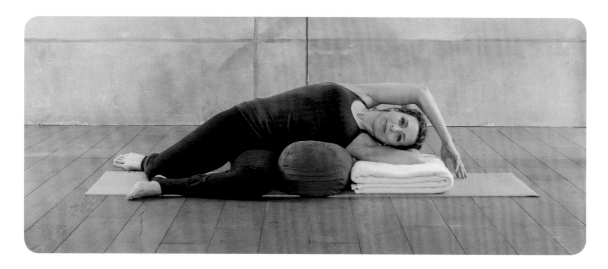

❀ **Lying Butterfly** (Supta Baddha Konasana)

This exercise opens your pelvic area, has a positive effect on the organs of the lower abdomen, and stretches the insides of the legs. It also expands your chest area, which can help you with deep breathing.

Effect

With Lying Butterfly the focus is on the meridians of the liver, kidneys, and spleen, and—when the arms are outstretched—on the lungs, heart, and pericardium meridians as well.

Practicing the exercise

Lie back on the mat; place a yoga block under your head, and a second one at shoulder height under your thoracic spine. Alternatively, you can use a soft cushion under your head. Bring the soles of your feet together, and let your knees sink outwards slowly. Should the stretch be too intense on the insides of the legs or the groin, you can place more blocks or cushions under your knees. Stretch the arms out long next to your head, and place them on the floor so that you can feel a stretch in the chest and shoulder area. If your fingertips go numb doing this or you do not have the range of motion to do this, change the position of the arms so that the hands are more at your side or on your stomach.

Stay in the position for three to five minutes. Take the arms back next to your body, close your legs, and push yourself up with an activated pelvic floor. Place the props to one side and relax into Supine Position (see page 87).

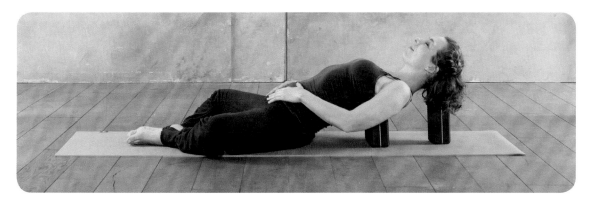

Lying Half Moon

In this position, the side stomach organs—the liver and spleen, the ascending and descending large intestine, and the lobe of the lung—are stretched on one side, and compressed on the other side.

Effect

Lying Half Moon works on the meridians of the gallbladder, small intestine, large intestine, and the triple warmer.

Practicing the exercise

Lie on your back and take your arms back onto the floor next to your head. With the left hand, you now grip the right wrist and move it away from the upper body to the left, little by little. Then push your legs slowly to the left, so that your body now takes on the shape of a lying half-moon and you feel the stretch on the right side of your body. Leave your feet parallel, or cross them. Take care that the pelvis remains on the floor and you do not tip to one side, so you will not lose the side stretch. The neck should remain relaxed.

Hold the position for three to five minutes, then come back to the center and change sides. Now relax into Supine Position (see page 87).

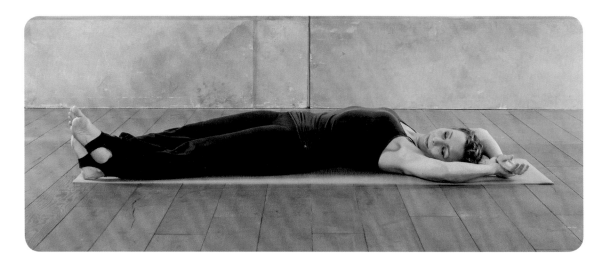

❋ Neck stretches

You can do these exercises daily if you have tension in the shoulder and neck area. They have a beneficial effect and release tension gently and effectively.

Effect

With the neck stretches, the focus is on the meridians of the bladder, gallbladder, stomach, small intestine, large intestine, and triple warmer; however, these are only stretched to a minor extent.

Practicing the exercise

1. Forward bend: sit comfortably on the floor or on a chair with a straight back. On the floor you can come into the cross-legged position, for example. First let your head sink forward dynamically . . .

2. Backbend: . . . and then gently backwards.

3. Sideways bend: now tilt the head to one side, as if you wanted to pull your upper ear upwards. Hold the position for a few breaths and change sides.

4. Rotation: now look alternately from side to side over both shoulders, and lengthen your neck while doing this. Finish with a sideways movement, where you lower your chin towards the collarbone and swing your head gently from side to side. Come back to the center and repeat the process on the other side, feeling into the neck and shoulder area.

Carry out as many repetitions as feels right to you.

(Stretches shown on next page)

Neck Stretches *(described on page 81)*

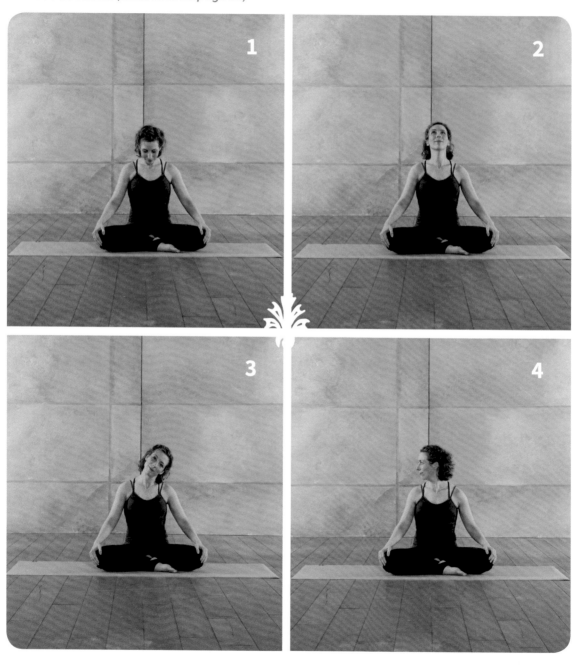

90-90 position (Deer)

In this position you open up the hip joints, once with an inner and once with an outer rotation. The opening of the hips is at its most intense if the legs are bent to an angle of 90 degrees, but it can also be a little gentler with less of a bend. The 90-90 position also stimulates the stomach organs.

Effect

The focus here is on the meridians of the gallbladder and bladder, and possibly also on the liver, kidneys, and spleen.

Practicing the exercise

1. Sit on the on the floor with your legs forming a 90-degree angle. That means the thigh of the right leg is pointing forward straight, and you bend the lower leg to a right angle. Take the left leg straight out to the side, and bend the lower leg into a right angle here, too. If this is not possible for you, you can also make the angle of the knee smaller, of course. Bend the upper body forward in a relaxed way. If necessary, use a blanket or bolster to support you.

2. Straighten up again for the **rotated** version: turn your upper body towards the right and now bend forward over the right thigh.

Remain in the position for three to five minutes, including the rotated version. Come back to the center, place both feet on the floor, and loosen your legs by moving them to and fro a few times. Repeat the exercise with the left leg forward. Then relax into Supine Position (see page 87).

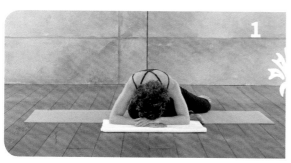
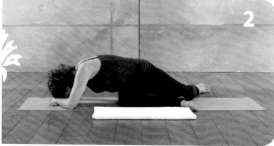

❦ Open Wings

This position opens the chest and stretches the front part of the shoulders. The muscles are often shortened in these areas due to daily poor posture—by sitting at the computer for hours, for example.

Effect

The focus is on the meridians of the lungs, heart, and pericardium.

Practicing the exercise

Start on your stomach and stretch your right arm out to the side at shoulder height, with the palm of your hand facing downwards. Now support yourself with your left arm and turn onto the right side of the body. Bend both knees and move your arm to a 90-degree angle from the body. Place a block or cushion under your head if the position of your neck feels uncomfortable. The further you lean your upper body back, the more intense the stretch gets. If you would like it to be a little softer, then lie on a folded blanket or keep the upper body further forward. You can also vary the angle of the arm, of course.

Stay in the position for two to three minutes, then come back onto your stomach and change sides. Relax in Resting Forward Pose (see page 88).

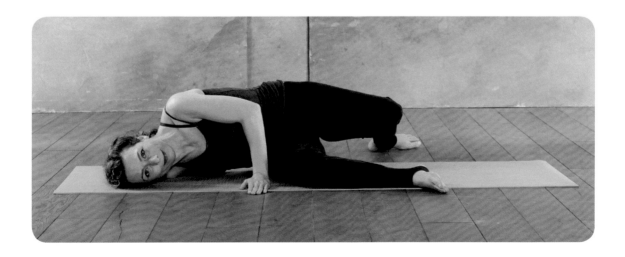

❦ **Quarter Dog** (Anahatasana)

This position stretches the front side of the body and the arms, and stimulates the stomach organs as well. It also expands the lobes of the lungs and therefore supports deep breathing.

Effect

Quarter Dog has an effect on the meridians of the stomach, spleen, kidneys, liver, bladder, lungs, and heart, and the pericardium in particular.

Practicing the exercise

1. Go onto all fours, taking your hands as far forward as possible. Your knees and pelvis are at the same height, and your hands are placed clearly in front of your shoulders. Let your breastbone sink passively towards the floor, and push your coccyx up actively. Place your forehead on the floor or on a blanket, and direct your breath to your back.

2. As a variation, you can also carry out this position with a **rotation**. Stretch your right arm out long, and take the left arm through and under the right one. Turn your head to the right, and place it to the side on the ground to relax into the rotated position. Then change sides.

Stay in the position for three to five minutes, including the right and left rotation. Let your buttocks release by sinking to the heels, and take your arms next to the legs so that you go into Child's Pose (see page 57).

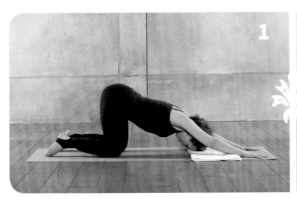
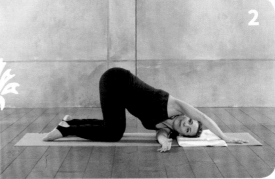

❧ **Rainbow Bridge** (Urdhva Dhanurasana)

This position mobilizes the thoracic spine, opens the heart chamber, and stretches the shoulders and insides of the arms.

Effect

The stretch is particularly effective on the meridians of the stomach, spleen, kidneys, liver, lungs, heart, and pericardium.

Practicing the exercise

Place a yoga bolster and a rolled-up blanket straight across the mat. Then lie down with your back on the bolster, which supports your pelvis and lumbar spine. Your shoulder blades are on the blanket, and your arms are placed alongside your head. If you would like to intensify the stretch, you can extend out your legs, or for a gentler variant, leave your feet placed on the floor.

Stay in Rainbow Bridge for three to five minutes. Then either sit up again with activated pelvic floor muscles, or roll to one side out of the position. Then relax into Supine Position (see page 87).

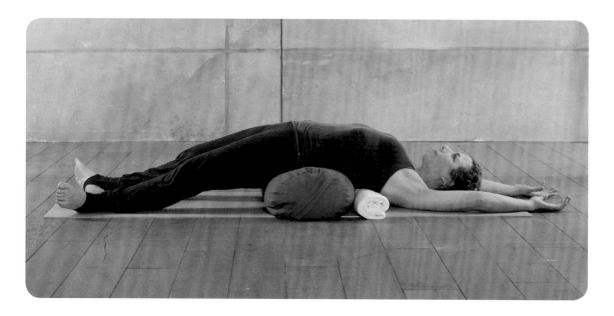

✤ **Relaxed Supine Position** (Shavasana, Pentacle)

Always carry out this position at the end of your practice, even if you may not think it is important. This gives your body time to bring the activated energies into unison and harmony, which is important for unfolding your capacity for self-healing. Beyond this, I recommend Relaxed Supine Position for neutralizing and relaxing into exercises in between.

Effect

The position does not have any special meridian effect, but supports the flow of energy in general.

Practicing the exercise

Lie on your back, with your arms a comfortable distance from the upper body so that you can breathe easily. Open your feet slightly and let the legs fall loosely to the side. Your head should be centered, and you can place it on a small cushion if this is more comfortable. Relax your whole body and give your weight to the floor. Keep your breathing calm and also try to let your mind be quiet. If you wish, you can run through your body in your mind, from bottom to top, and make contact with each individual area. Start with the feet, then move to the legs, then the pelvis, the spine, the entire back, the abdomen, the chest area, the shoulders, the arms, and the hands. Also relax the throat and neck area, and the face. Then relax your whole body consciously once again.

After a quiet Yin sequence, the final relaxation can be shorter than after a strenuous Yang sequence. Five to ten minutes in the position will probably be enough. One or two minutes in Relaxed Supine Position is optimal between two exercises, before you move into the next position.

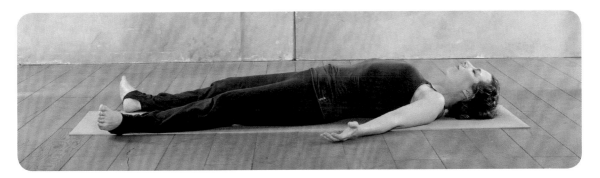

❀ **Resting Forward Pose** (Adhvasana)

Resting Forward Pose is recommended after positions in which the front side of your body is directed towards the floor.

Effect

The position has no particular effect on the meridians, but supports the flow of energy in general.

Practicing the exercise

Lie on your stomach and rest your head comfortably on your hands—looking downwards, or with your head turned in a relaxed way to the side. Your feet are slightly open, and the heels go towards one another or outwards, depending on your hip joint anatomy.

Remain in the position as long as it feels comfortable. Draw your hands and the balls of your feet up again. You can then also spend some time in Child's Pose (see page 57).

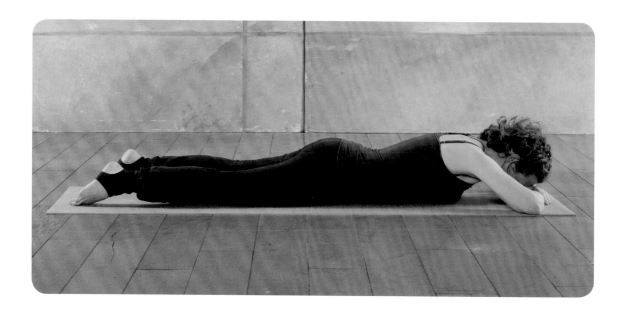

❧ Resting Pose

Resting Pose is a very beneficial position for the back, especially after exercises that involve strong back bends, such as Saddle (see page 90). It releases the sacral-iliac joint, and has a very relaxing effect if the hands are in contact with the third eye chakra. It is therefore very good to do this prior to meditation, or before the final relaxation at the end.

Effect

Resting Pose has no special effect on the meridians, but supports the flow of energy in general.

Practicing the exercise

Lie on your back, bend the legs, and open your feet more than hip width. Let the knees fall towards one another. Put the hands together into Prayer Pose, and place either the thumbs or fingertips on your third eye chakra (see page 27).

Stay in the position as long as it feels good. Pull the knees up to release, and either rock upwards or come into the sitting position from your side.

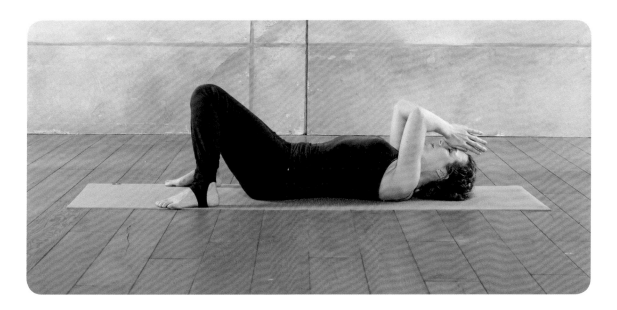

❦ **Saddle** (Supta Virasana)

This position stretches the front side of the body from the thighs to the shoulders, and also stimulates the stomach organs. It gently compresses the spine as well, which can activate the production of bone tissue. It is a key position in Yin Yoga, as it works on the entire spine in the backbend as well as the long fascia chains on the front side of the body. It also focuses on the lordosis of the spine. Many find Saddle one of the most challenging exercises in Yin Yoga practice; it can be made considerably gentler by using props.

Effect

Saddle harmonizes the meridians of the stomach, spleen, liver, and kidneys, and with outstretched arms, works on the meridians of the lungs, heart, and pericardium as well.

Practicing the exercise

1. Place a yoga bolster lengthways on the mat and sit in front of the bolster—either in the Ankle Stretch (that is, with the buttocks touching your heels), or in Hero, where you come into a sitting position with the buttocks between your lower legs. If this sitting position causes pressure in the knees, you can also sit on a yoga block. If there is a lot of tension in the bridge of the foot, place two small rolled-up hand towels under the ankles, or cushion the bridge of the foot using a blanket. Now lie back on the bolster, your arms comfortably behind your head. If you still find the position too difficult, then place the bolster a little higher by putting a cushion or blanket (for example) underneath or on top of it.

2. If you would like to feel the position more intensely, you can take away all the props and carry out Saddle directly on the mat.

3. To start with, you can also do **Half Saddle**. For this, bend just one leg in the Ankle Stretch or Hero, and extend the other leg out or place your foot in front of you. If you tip too far to the side, then place a block under the side of the buttocks where you feel the imbalance. As in Saddle, you can also use the bolster here, of course.

Remain in the position for three to five minutes; for Half Saddle, remember to change sides. Sit up straight again with an activated pelvic floor, and then come into Child's Pose (see page 57) or relax into Supine Position (see page 87).

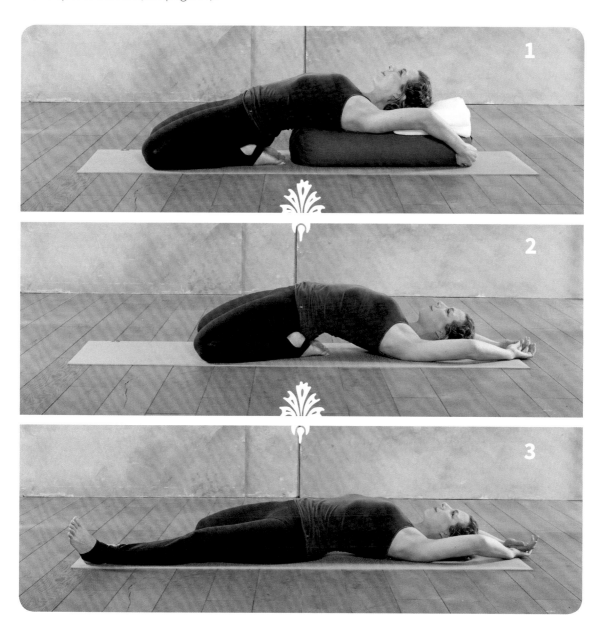

❦ **Seagrass** (Viparita Karani)

The gentle inversion of this position stimulates the stomach organs and cardiovascular system. It is also a particularly good release for the legs.

Effect

Seagrass does not place so much focus on stretching the meridians, but on the relaxing effect.

Practicing the exercise

Place a yoga bolster or rolled-up blanket straight across the mat and lie on it. Place your upper body behind it to bring the pelvis into a raised position. Stretch the legs upwards, and find the point where you can hold it effortlessly. Take your arms back slowly and place them next to your head. During menstruation, you can also assume the position without raising the pelvis. For a more intensive version, let the legs drop back slightly more towards the floor (I do not recommend this version if you have issues in your cervical spine).

Stay in this gentle exercise for five minutes or more. Then bend the legs again, draw your knees to your chest, and roll sideways out of the position. Relax into Supine Position (see page 87).

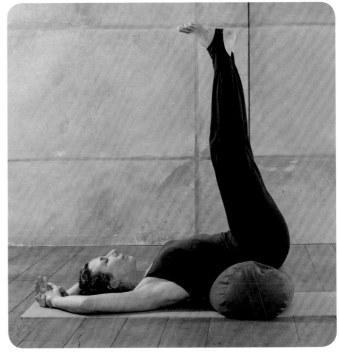

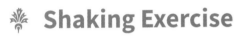 Shaking Exercise

This exercise releases tension and has a vitalizing effect at the same time. Many Asians practice it daily for up to twenty minutes as preventive healthcare.

Effect

Shaking Exercise stimulates the entire flow of the Chi. Used Chi flows down into the meridians and is deposited into the ground via the feet, where it can be neutralized once again.

Practicing the exercise

Stand up straight, open the feet to around shoulder width, and let your arms hang loosely. Let your body remain soft and open. Now start seesawing movements from the knees. Let the impulse run through your entire body and, if you like, gradually start shaking more vigorously. You can also keep to the gentle version, if you wish. If possible, increase the length of your exhalations to channel out the used Chi more effectively.

Shake your body as long as it feels right. Then relax into a resting standing position for a few breaths.

❦ **Shoelace** (Gomukhasana)

This position mobilizes the lumbar spine area and opens up the hips. Both sides may feel completely different, as there are small differences in the hip joints in most people. It also stretches the outer thigh fascia, which is naturally rather tight. This stretch therefore often feels tougher than positions that tend to focus on the insides of the thighs, but it can be easily helped by using props. Furthermore, Shoelace massages the organs of the stomach via the forward bend, and thus can stimulate the metabolism.

Effect

Shoelace works on the meridians of the gallbladder and bladder, and possibly on the liver, kidneys, and spleen. With the shoulder stretch version, it also stimulates the small intestine, large intestine, and triple warmer meridians.

Practicing the exercise

1. Sit on the floor or on a folded blanket, and cross your right leg over the left one in such a way that your knees are one above the other. If this position causes pain in the knees, or your hip joints do not allow this, then stretch the left leg out in front of you, or sit lengthways on a yoga bolster so that your knees are supported. You can also cushion the area surface supporting your knees with a small blanket or towel to avoid painful pressure. Now let your upper body sink forward with a rounded back, and place your hands loosely on the right knee, on a prop, or on the floor.

2. For an additional **shoulder stretch**, you can work with a block in this position, which you place in front of the knees. Bend your elbows, and position the left upper arm in the crook of the right arm. Relax your upper body and let yourself sink forward towards the block with a rounded back. Alternatively, you can also place your arms crossed on your knees.

3. Straighten up again slowly and now come into a **side bend**. Put your left hand to the side next to your left foot, and tilt the upper body leftwards. Take your right arm and stretch it above your head.

4. You can then combine Shoelace with a **rotation**. Straighten your spine and place the left hand on the outside of the right knee. Take your right hand behind your pelvis and turn to the right, keeping your spine straight.

It is up to you whether you do Shoelace with or without a shoulder stretch. Remain in the position for three to five minutes, including the side bend to the left and the rotation to the right. Then come back to the center, stretch your legs out long in front of you, and move to and fro a few times. Now change sides and do the position with the left leg above, and in doing so tilt right and turn left. Alternatively, you can also stay in the forward bend. Finally, stretch your legs and relax into Supine Position (see page 87).

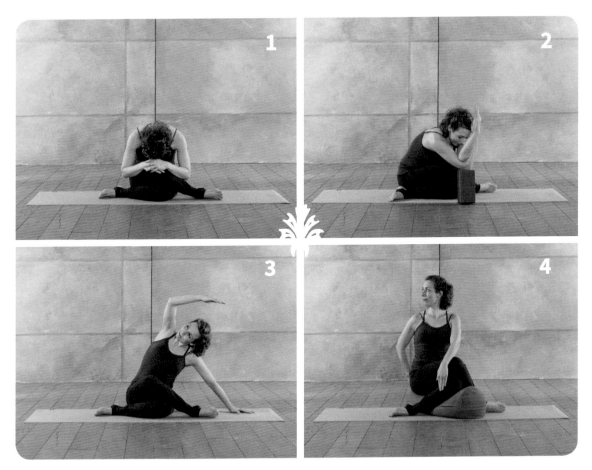

❀ **Sitting Twisted Roots** (Jathara Parivartanasana)

This position gently massages and mobilizes the spine.

Effect

Sitting Twisted Roots works on the meridians of the bladder and gallbladder.

Practicing the exercise

Place a yoga bolster or a rolled-up blanket lengthways on the mat, and sit left of it on the floor. If you would like to integrate a little more opening of the hips, bend your legs comfortably to the left, at 90 degrees to the ankle if you wish. Place your fingers on the floor and press them in to create length in the spine. Now rotate your upper body to the right and lie relaxed on the bolster. Bend the arms and place your head in such a way that you are looking to the left. If this is too intense for your cervical spine, then keep the head in the middle or look to the right. Direct your breath gently towards the abdomen.

Hold the position for three to five minutes, push yourself up again, and change sides. Then place the props to the side and relax into Resting Forward Pose (see page 88) or go into Relaxed Supine Position (see page 87).

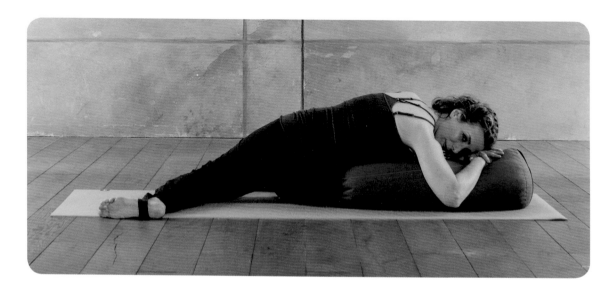

❁ **Sleeping Swan** (Eka Pada Raja Kapotanasana)

This position opens up the hips and has a relaxing effect on the lower back. In the rotation, it also stretches the upper body.

Effect

Sleeping Swan works on the meridians of the gallbladder and bladder. In the rotation, it also stimulates the small intestine meridian, the large intestine meridian, and the triple warmer meridian.

Practicing the exercise

1. Come onto all fours and pull your right knee forward to the right wrist. Bend the leg in such a way that your foot points to the left side and you can place the outside of the leg on the floor. For a greater opening of the hips, bring the upper and lower leg into a 90-degree angle, and if that feels difficult to you, make the angle smaller accordingly. If this position causes pain in the knees or if possible lack of balance on either side of the body is uncomfortable, sit higher, perhaps with buttocks and knees on a yoga bolster positioned lengthways. Your back leg remains long on the floor. Now place your upper body relaxed on the bent leg, and rest your head in your hands or on a yoga bolster.

2. For a side stretch, you can include a slight **rotation**. Walk your arms rightwards, bit by bit, on the outside of the bent leg until you feel a pleasant stretch on the left side of the upper body.

Remain in the position for three to five minutes, including the side rotation. Alternatively, you can also stay in the bent-forward position. Straighten up again, come into Downward Facing Dog (see page 115), and then change sides. Now relax and neutralize by going into Supine Position (see page 87) or Child's Pose (see page 57).

(Pose shown on next page)

Sleeping Swan *(described on page 97)*

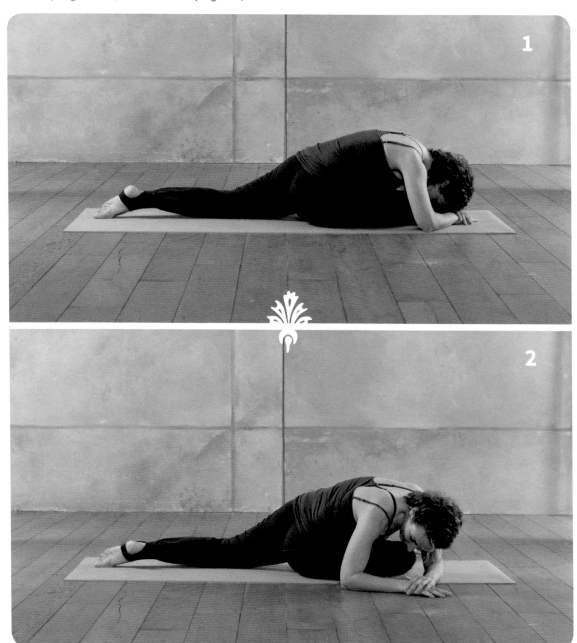

✿ Sphinx (Bhujangasana) **and Seal** (Urdhva Mukha Svanasana)

This position opens up the chest, stretches and stimulates the stomach organs, and gently compresses the kidneys.

Effect

The focus is on the meridians of the stomach, spleen, kidney, and liver. The shoulder-stretch version also focuses on the small intestine, large intestine, and triple warmer meridians.

Practicing the exercise

1. Lie on your stomach, place your forearms on the floor, and straighten your upper body. For a gentle version of the **Sphinx**, which supports you when releasing in this position, you can place a yoga bolster or rolled-up blanket straight across the mat underneath your ribcage.

2. For an additional **shoulder stretch**, cross your arms in front of the body. Bend the elbows, place the right upper arm in the crook of the left arm, and support the crossed elbow; if you wish, you can also use a blanket or two blocks. Rest your head on your arms and let yourself sink forward passively into the stretch. You can then also change the position of your arms.

3. For more of a backbend, prop yourself up on your hands and push up your upper body, using your arms, to come into **Seal**. Breathe out deeply and let yourself sink down into the spine, as in a hanging bridge. You can leave your legs slightly open to release the lumbar spine.

If you would like to do a slightly stronger backbend, then bend the knees so that the soles of the feet are facing the floor. During pregnancy, it is better to work with two yoga bolsters; these are placed above and below the stomach to avoid any pressure in the belly. Remain in Sphinx for three to five minutes, including the shoulder stretch, or in Seal. Release the position and rock the pelvis to and fro a little. Then relax into Supine Position (see page 87). For pregnant women, Child's Pose (see page 57) with open legs is recommended.

(Poses shown on next page)

Sphinx and Seal *(described on page 99)*

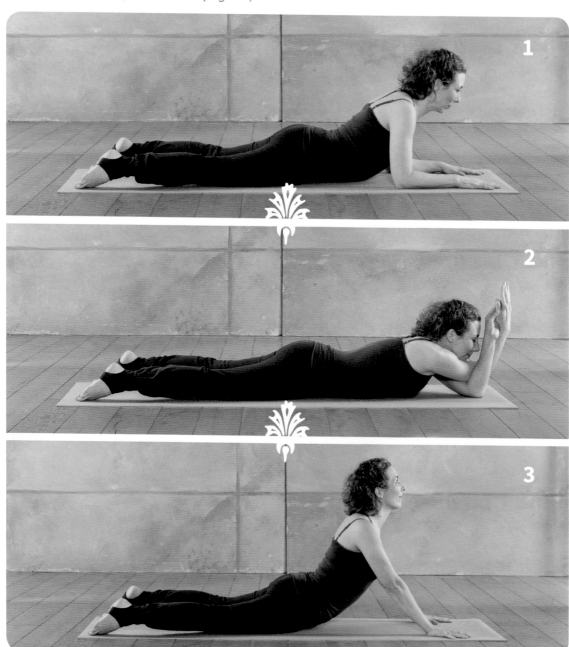

❦ **Square** (Agnisthambasana)

This position opens up the hip joints, stretches the lower back, and mobilizes the spine. It also stretches the outer thigh fascia, which are naturally rather tight. Therefore, many people find this stretch much harder than the hip opener, which tends to focus on the insides of the legs.

Effect

Square stimulates the meridians of the gallbladder and bladder, and possibly also the liver and the kidney meridian. In the rotation and the side bend, it has an increased effect on the gallbladder meridian, and the side bend also effects the meridians of the small intestine, large intestine, and triple warmer.

Practicing the exercise

1. Come into a cross-legged position, and place a cushion under the buttocks if necessary. If your hip joints allow the opening, then position your left lower leg parallel to the front edge of the mat and place your right lower leg flush over it. If you experience an unpleasant feeling in the knee doing this, you can also place your right foot lower and put it on the lower leg, or remain in the cross-legged position. Support your right knee with a cushion if you wish. Now put the palms of your hands together, place the forearms on your legs, bend the upper body forward in a relaxed way, and lower your head. Alternatively, you can rest your arms or hands on the floor or on a support. In addition to the stretch, you can also activate the powerful Liver 3 **acupressure point**, a point on the liver meridian, which is a thumb width between the large toe and second toe, in an indentation in the bridge of the foot. It mobilizes the blocked liver energy and calms the liver and mind. The stimulation also encourages the flow of the Chi and the blood flow throughout the entire body. Press this point as long and as firmly as feels comfortable. If you are pregnant, you should only hold it very gently.

2. For an even gentler version, you can also **cross your lower legs** classically and support your knees with two yoga blocks, for example. Place your hands to the side next to your knees, and then bend forward with a rounded back and relaxed neck.

3. Sit straight again to combine Square with a **side bend**. Place your left hand to the side next to you and tilt your upper body to the left side. Take the right arm next to your head or leave it behind your back.

4. Return to the center and now finish with a **rotation**. Place your left hand on your right knee, support yourself with your right hand behind your pelvis, and turn right with a straight spine.

Stay in the position for three to five minutes, including the side bend to the left and the rotation to the right. Release and loosen your legs, then cross the lower legs the other way around and repeat the exercise, with the side bend to the right and the rotation to the left. Alternatively, you can simply remain in the forward bend.

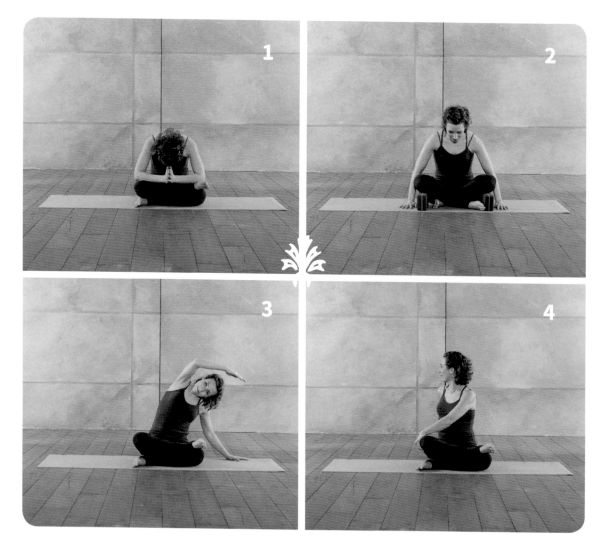

❀ Squat (Malasana)

Squat has a detoxifying effect on the body, as it massages and stimulates the intestine and ensures good digestion. The position also strengthens the ankles, mobilizes the knee and hip joints, and stretches the buttocks and lumbar spine.

Effect

The squat mainly has an effect on the meridians of the liver, kidneys, spleen, and bladder.

Practicing the exercise

Position yourself with slightly straddled legs, your toes pointing outwards or straight in front. Now slowly bend the knees and lower your buttocks towards the floor until the calves and thighs are touching. Should your heels be lifted from the floor in the lowered position, then place a rolled-up blanket under them to find a good balance. If you find Squat too tough on your knees, you can place a few blocks or a yoga bolster under your buttocks, or sit directly on the floor with your legs still bent. Put your hands into Prayer Pose, place the tips of your fingers on the third eye chakra (see page 27), and bend forward with your back relaxed. In the position, you can either stay quite still or include gentle rocking movements back and forth. For an additional stretch in the neck, fold your hands behind your head and stretch gently here.

Remain in Squat for three to five minutes. To release, stretch the legs slowly and come into the counter-position in a standing forward bend (see page 60).

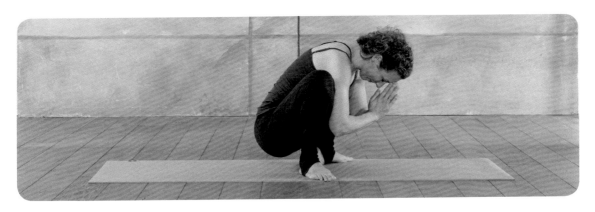

❧ **Turtle** (Kurmasana)

This position opens up the hips and stretches the lower back. Opening the pelvis wide can have a regulating effect on the organs of the abdomen.

Effect

Turtle works on the meridians of the liver, kidneys, spleen, gallbladder, and bladder.

Practicing the exercise

1. Sit on the mat and place the soles of your feet together. The feet are far enough from the pelvis that the legs form a diamond shape. Tilt forward in the upper body, and feed the arms through your lower legs so that you can clasp your feet. Let your back become as round as the shell of a turtle. Take your attention inwards, just like a turtle going back into its shell.

2. In this position you can also stimulate the Kidney 3 **acupressure point** to help build up energy in the kidneys and counter exhaustion, menstrual disorders, and pain in the lower back. It is located between the ankle and the Achilles tendon on the inside of the leg. Note: this point is not recommended for pregnant women.

Remain in Turtle for three to five minutes, and you can stimulate the acupressure point as long as it feels comfortable. Then roll upwards again slowly and relax into Supine Position (see page 87).

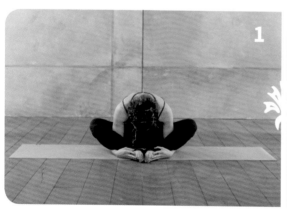 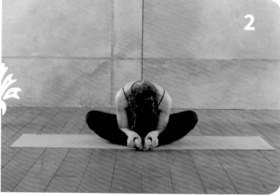

Twisted Arms

This position stretches the arms and shoulders, and mobilizes the entire shoulder girdle. Like Embracing Wings (see page 67), it is one of the few Yin Yoga exercises that reaches the outsides of the arms and the meridians that run through them.

Effect

Twisted Arms has a particular effect on the small intestine, large intestine, and triple warmer.

Practicing the exercise

Lie on your back and shift your weight to the left side so that you can angle your right arm behind your back. Turn backwards and place yourself on the angled arm. You can place the left arm to the side or stretched out upwards. Breathe calmly into your stomach. Please take care that the tips of your fingers do not go numb; if they do, then you should change the position, by placing your head higher, for example, or moving your extended arms a few centimeters upwards or downwards.

Remain in the position for two to three minutes. Turn to the left a little so that you can release your arms and change sides. Then relax into Supine Position (see page 87).

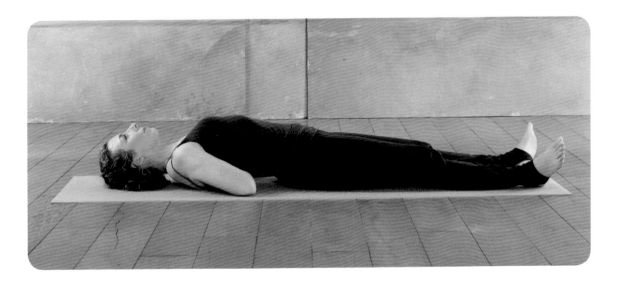

❀ **Twisted Roots** (Jathara Parivartanasana)

The position stimulates the stomach organs through stretching and breathing. I find it one of the most healing exercises there is in yoga for back complaints, as it keeps the spine and surrounding fascial tissues elastic and supple. It can be used preventively, but also is useful, in acute cases, if there is sufficient support under the legs. The Twisted Roots is highly suitable for concluding a series of exercises, as it closes the pelvis again and therefore keeps the energy in the chakras more efficiently.

Effect

Twisted Roots mainly works on the meridians of the gallbladder, bladder, lungs, heart, and pericardium.

Practicing the exercise

1. Lie on your back, pull your knees up to your chest, and let your bent legs sink onto the floor to the left. You can place your arms to the side at shoulder height, or stretch them out on the floor above you. Look towards your right hand if you want to include a rotation in the cervical spine. Give all your weight to the floor and breathe into your stomach to intensify the massaging effect on your stomach organs.

2. If you want to **intensify the stretch**, you can try the following versions. Start by lying on your back, place your feet hip-width apart on the mat, and let your knees fall to the side as described above. Now release the lower foot from the floor and place it on the outside of the upper leg or on the knee.

3. Besides the rotation, with Twisted Roots you can also **intensify the rotation**. To do this, lying on your back, stretch out the left leg and place the right foot on leg. From here, let your right knee sink left to the floor, with a prop underneath if required. You feel the effect even more intensively if you place your left hand on the right thigh.

Stay in the selected position for three to five minutes. Then come back to the center, grip your knees and press them briefly to your chest, rock to and fro a few times, and then change sides.

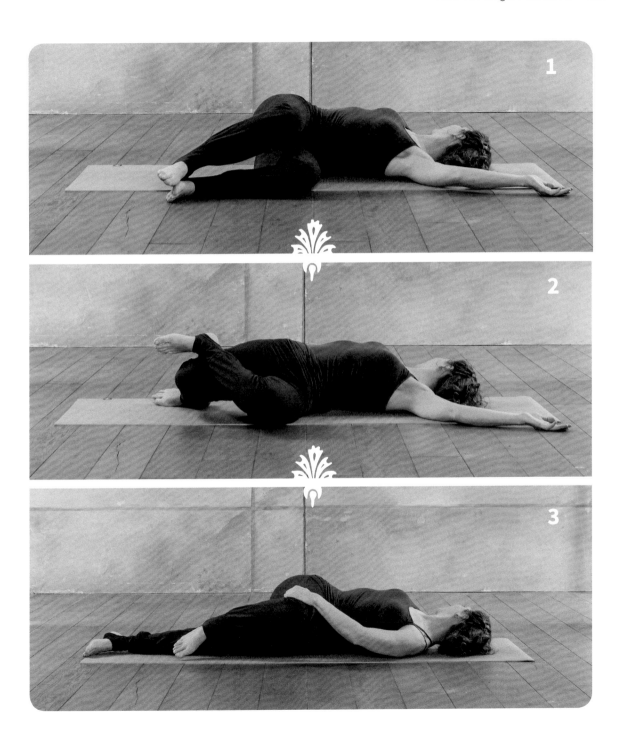

❧ Twisted Roots Heart Opener
(Jathara Parivartanasana)

This exercise opens up the chest and shoulders, mobilizes the spine, and stretches the sides of the body.

Effect

Twisted Roots Heart Opener has an effect on the meridians of the gallbladder, spleen, stomach, kidneys, liver, lungs, heart, and pericardium.

Practicing the exercise

Roll up a blanket or towel to form a small bolster and place it straight across the mat. Lie down on your back so that the bolster is underneath your shoulder blades. Open your feet out to hip width and let your knees sink to the left side. Take the arms back onto the floor next to your head and tilt your head to the side, keeping it relaxed. For a gentler version, you can also place a yoga bolster under your lower leg; for more stretch, release the lower foot and place it on the outside of the upper leg.

Remain in the position for three to five minutes. To release, come into Folded Pose (see page 117), sway to and fro a few times, and then change sides. Finally, place the bolster to one side and relax into Supine Position (see page 87).

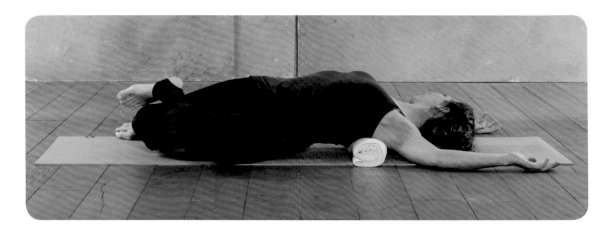

❋ Twisted Twisted Roots
(Jathara Parivartanasana)

In this position, the organs of the stomach are stimulated by the twist. It also mobilizes the spine and stretches the surrounding fascia.

Effect

Twisted Twisted Roots mainly works on the meridians of the gallbladder, bladder, lungs, heart, and pericardium.

Practicing the exercise

Lie on your back and place your feet on the floor. Cross your legs as you would if sitting on a chair. Stretch your arms out long next to your head and let your crossed legs fall to the left side. Look to the right, if you would like to include the rotation in the cervical spine. Bring the knees back to the center, leave the legs in the position, and now place them to the right. Come back to the middle again and pull your knees to your chest. Raise your head and stay in Folded Pose (see page 117) for a short while. Lie flat again, cross your legs the other way, and repeat the process.

Remain in the position for three to five minutes and then change the position of the legs. To finish, relax into Supine Position (see page 87).

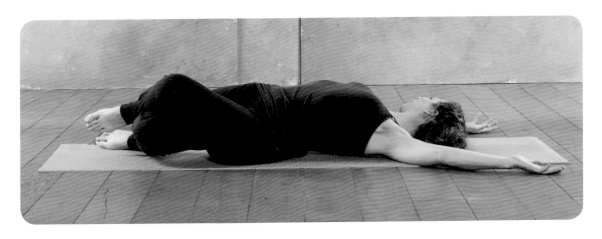

❋ The **Yang Yoga Positions**

These exercises are intended to bring heat or Yang energy into your body between poses, if you notice you have cooled down a lot or if you are becoming too tired. You can carry them out between the Yin exercises anytime. Hold the positions for between five to eight breaths—or for more, or fewer if you wish. As the effect is not as great with the short power exercises as with those you hold longer for the Yin exercises, you will not find any details on the effects on the individual meridians here.

❈ Active Bridge (Setu Bandha Sarvangasana)

Bridge stretches the front side and strengthens the rear side of the body. The lobes of the lungs expand, which can have a positive effect on deep breathing.

Practicing the exercise

Lie on your back and place the feet hip-width apart. Raise your pelvis slightly and grip your hands together under your buttocks. Bring the shoulders and upper arms closer together and push your pelvis straight up. Either hold the position statically, or do it dynamically by lowering the buttocks when exhaling and then inhaling again when you rise.

Remain in the positon for five to eight breaths. Roll your spine back to the floor disc by disc, and to balance it out come into Folded Pose (see page 117).

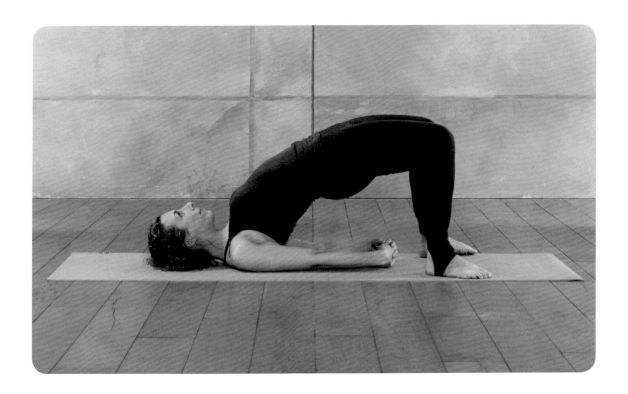

❀ **Boat** (Paripurna Navasana)

This position strengthens the core, the back, and the legs. It also promotes a sense of balance, and produces Yang energy in the form of heat in the body. You can also build this exercise into your sequence if you practice many forward bends and you have stretched the spine a great deal in doing so. It will tighten the muscles again and has a balancing effect.

Practicing the exercise

1. Sit on the mat, lean your upper body back slightly with a straight back, and at the same time lift your lower thighs with legs bent so that they are parallel to the floor. Activate your pelvic floor, look straight ahead, and stretch the arms forward at shoulder height.

2. You can either hold it statically, or go into a dynamic version. To do this, stretch your legs out long, and lean your upper body further back while breathing in; on the exhale, come back upwards. Feel free to experiment with your breath here. It may possibly be better for you the other way around. If you are not yet familiar with this position, it can be quite strenuous to start with. Take a slow and cautious approach to this strength exercise.

Remain in the position for five to eight breaths. You can then relax for a moment in Coachman (see page 51).

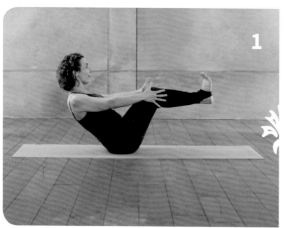
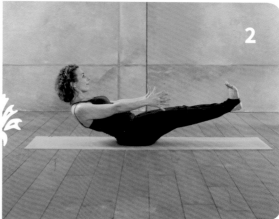

❀ **Camel** (Ustrasana)

This exercise strengthens the rear side of the body and stretches the front side. It is ideal to pre-pare for Saddle (see page 90).

Practicing the exercise

Come into a knee stand. Your upper body is straight and your legs are hip-width apart. (If you gen-erally have sensitive knees, or the pressure suddenly feels unpleasant, you can cushion your knees with a soft blanket.) Then push your pelvis and thighs forward and bend your spine backwards in the chest area. Stretch your arms and support yourself on your ankles using your hands.

Either hold the position statically, or do it dynamically by straightening up on the inhale and lowering your buttocks again on the exhale. As it is a Yang position, you should avoid having a very hollow back, and don't hold the tension in your neck. If your spine does not allow the opening, you can "lengthen" your arms by putting blocks under your hands. If you have neck problems, the cervi-cal spine should stay long in the back bend.

Remain in the position for five to eight breaths and then relax into Child's Pose (see page 57).

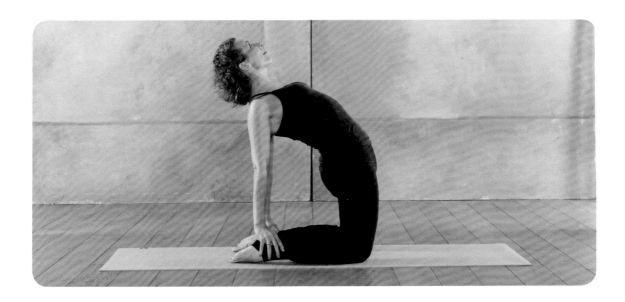

Cat and Cow (Chakravakasana)

This sequence of exercises gently mobilizes the spine and has a balancing effect on the upper body.

Practicing the exercise

1. Come onto all fours and move your spine gently up and down. If you cannot kneel on the floor, move the spine while standing. While exhaling, let your back become very rounded, like a cat arching its back. Open the shoulder blades and look towards your navel.

2. Now push the spine gently downwards again, and while inhaling, let your back drop like a hanging bridge. Pull your shoulder blades together and look upwards.

Repeat this five to eight times. Allow it to be a gentle and dynamic exercise. Then come into Child's Pose (see page 57) and relax the spine.

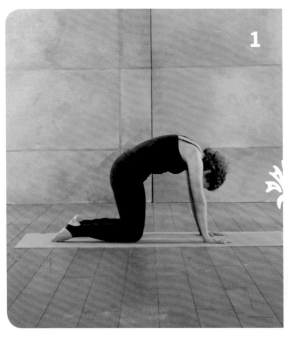
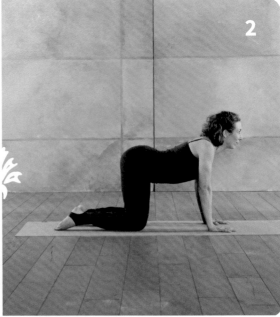

❧ **Downward Facing Dog** (Adho Mukha Svanasana)

In this position, the entire back of the body is stretched; it also strengthens the front side of the body and arms. Downward Facing Dog is a gentle inverted position that is very good for helping relieve backache, tense shoulders, and shortened backs of the thighs.

Practicing the exercise

Come onto all fours, with your hands below your shoulders and knees under your pelvis. Then stretch your legs, and relax your head between your arms so that your body forms an inverted V. If this feels difficult or uncomfortable, then bend your legs or shift your hands or feet a little. For a more intense version, you can stretch out one leg behind when inhaling, hold it for a few breaths, and lower it again when exhaling. Raise and lower the right and left leg alternately.

Remain in the position for five to eight breaths. Then come back onto your knees and stay in Child's Pose (see page 57).

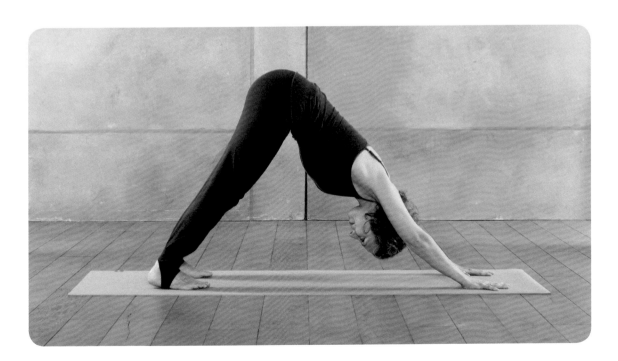

❀ **Dynamic Windshield Wiper** (Jathara Parivartanasana)

This exercise loosens the hip joints and relaxes the lower back. It is an ideal neutral pose to use after poses that open up the hips. It can be done lying down or with the lower arms drawn up, and is also good to do in between exercises to relax the back and neutralize the hip joints without building up heat. You can also practice it a few times before you go on to Twisted Roots Heart Opener (see page 108).

Practicing the exercise

Lie on your back and place the feet hip-width apart. Stretch your arms out long and let them rest, relaxed, next to your head. Then move your knees dynamically from one side to the other, just like a windshield wiper. If you wish, you can also support yourself on your lower arms and raise the upper body a little.

Move your legs to and fro a few times.

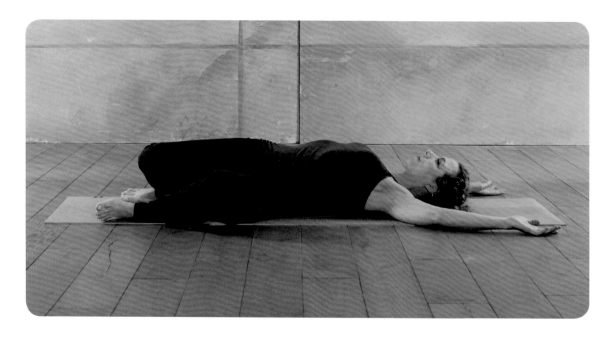

❀ **Folded Pose** (Apanasana)

This position gently stretches the spine, the entire back, and the neck. It also massages the abdominal organs, and is very good for neutralizing after intensive backbends. It can also be very beneficial for people who feel constricted in Child's Pose, or who experience a sense of pressure from this. In the rocking version, it is helpful for releasing the back in between poses.

Practicing the exercise

Lie on your back, bend the legs, and pull them towards the upper body. Place your arms around the lower legs to increase the pressure a little more. Keeping the legs either open or closed, raise your head off the floor and roll it slightly forward. If you wish, rock gently to and fro, or back and forth.

Remain in the position for five to eight breaths.

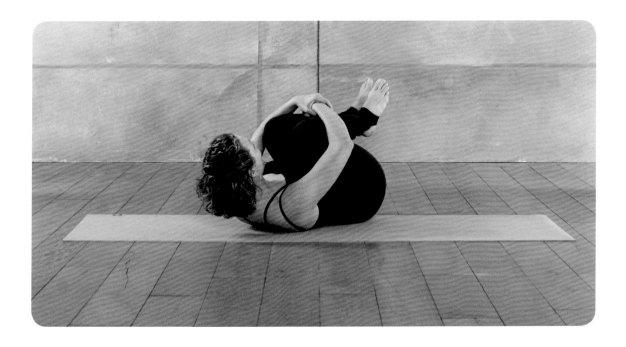

❧ **Hinge** (Urdhva Prasarita Padasana)

This exercise gives strength to the back and abdomen, and makes the hip flexors more powerful. It is balancing after many intensive forward bends.

Practicing the exercise

Lie on your back, place your feet on the floor, and put your hands under the lumbar spine or buttocks for stabilization. Now lift your head slightly from the floor and stretch your legs upwards vertically. Tighten the toes. Activate your pelvis and let your stretched legs (or, for less intensity, bent legs) sink slowly towards the floor. You can hold the position briefly just above the floor, or bring your legs directly upwards again.

Do three to five repetitions. Put your head on the floor again and lower the legs. To relax, you can also pull the knees to the chest, hug them, and rock them to and fro a few times.

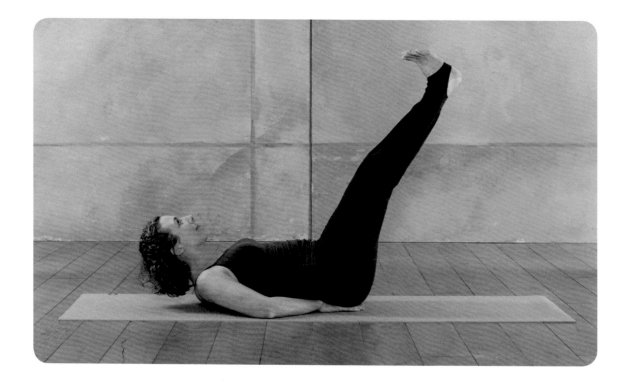

✤ **Infant** (Shalabasana)

This exercise strengthens the whole back and the buttock muscles. It stretches the front side of the upper body and massages the abdomen. It can also be used as a brief active exercise before passive backbends, or between positions with a forward bend.

Practicing the exercise

Lie on your front and place your arms outstretched behind you. Center the strength in your body, and then raise the upper body, arms, and legs at the same time. For more intensity, you can stretch the arms out in front. For a gentler version, leave the legs on the floor or just raise one leg and one arm diagonally.

Stay in the position for five to eight breaths. Then neutralize your back in Resting Forward Pose (see page 88), and move your pelvis gently back and forth a few times.

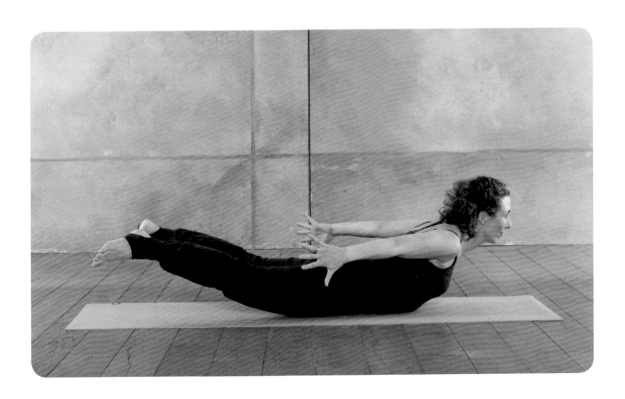

❋ **Plank** (Chaturanga Dandasana)

This position brings strength to the whole body and produces Yang energy in the form of heat. It strengthens the muscles in the arms and back strongly, and also activates core strength.

Practicing the exercise

1. Come onto all fours, with your hands under your shoulders and your knees under your pelvis. Now stretch your legs behind you, one after the other; go onto your toes, tense your core muscles, and hold your head as an elongation of your spine. Your spine should be in a straight line. Activate your core, hold the position, and let your breath continue to flow.

2. For a dynamic version, bend your arms far enough so that your body is just above the floor. When inhaling, push yourself back up. If you are not yet familiar with the exercise, it can be very strenuous to start with. If that is the case for you, challenge yourself gently with this strength exercise and begin with your knees on the ground.

Remain in this position for five to eight breaths. From here, come into Relaxed Supine Position (see page 87) or into Child's Pose (see page 57), and slowly calm your breathing again.

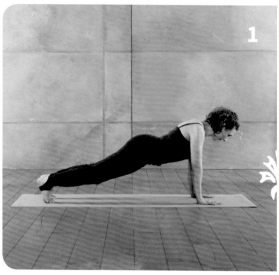
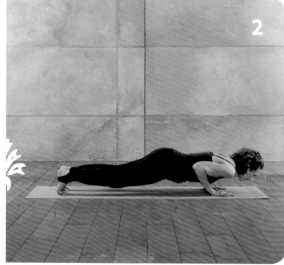

❋ **Tabletop** (Purvottanasana)

This exercise is like a reversed version of the push-up, and strengthens the whole body. The chest and shoulder area are also stretched.

Practicing the exercise

Sit on the mat, open your feet hip-width apart, and position your hands behind your back, with the fingertips pointing towards the buttocks. Bring strength into your body, and lift your pelvis far enough upwards that your legs and upper body form a straight line. Hold your neck with strength. Remain in the position statically, or do it dynamically by letting your buttocks sink when exhaling and raising them again when inhaling. Alternatively, you can also bend and extend the arms.

Remain in the position for five to eight breaths. Circle your wrists a few times in both directions to neutralize them, and come into Coachman for a few breaths (see page 51).

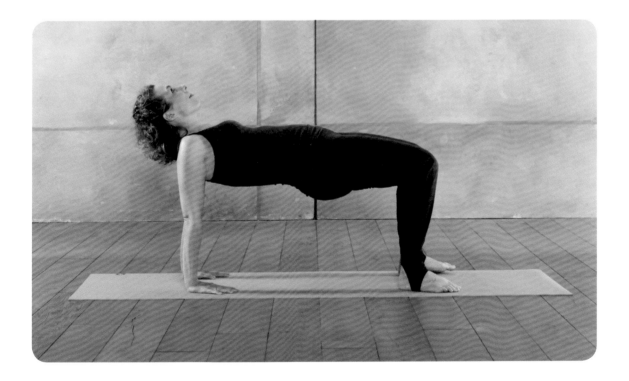

✤ **Tripod** (Camatkarasana)

This exercise strengthens the back and arms. It also stretches the shoulders and chest as well as the abdomen.

Practicing the exercise

Sit on the mat with outstretched legs. Place your left hand as support behind your pelvis, with your right foot on the floor and the left leg stretched out. Now press the three points of the left heel, the right foot, and the left hand to the floor and also raise your pelvis. Stretch the right arm to the ceiling, and either look upwards to your right hand or downwards to your left hand. Either hold the position statically, or practice it dynamically by letting your buttocks sink downwards again when exhaling and pushing upwards again when inhaling.

Hold the position for five to eight breaths and then change sides. Circle your wrist a few times in both directions.

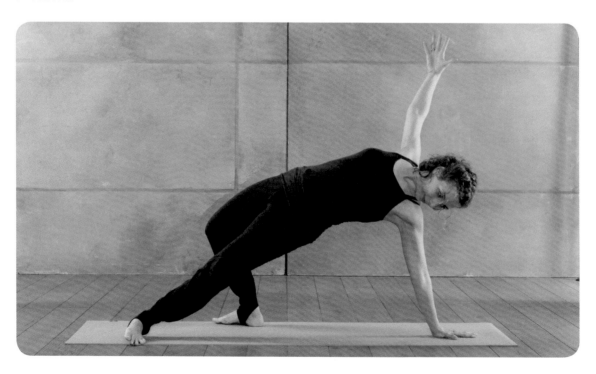

❧ The Healing **Breathing Techniques**

Breathing is our elixir of life—we could only survive without it for a few minutes. At the energetic level, consciously directed breathing techniques are a wonderful tool for connecting body and mind. As the breath is always in the present, these techniques are ideal for bringing peace of mind and reducing distracting thoughts. The selected exercises are all very gentle, and you can also practice them independently of the sequences—in stressful situations, for example, or in the evenings before going to sleep. The positive effect of conscious breathing will certainly become noticeable very quickly, even if you are not yet familiar with targeted breathing techniques and are practicing them for the first time.

❧ Four-Part Taoist Breath

You can try the Four-Part Taoist Breath all by itself, before or after practicing Yin Yoga. This breathing technique symbolizes the energy flow of Yin and Yang. It brings peace and relaxation and clears the mind. Practice it until you feel inner peace.

Practicing the exercise

1 and 2. Come into an Ankle or Toe Stretch, or alternatively into Easy Pose. Place the palms of your hands together and take the hands into Prayer Pose in front of your heart, breathing in. Now move the hands forward in slow motion when breathing out.

3 and 4. With your arms long, turn the palms upwards and start to roll up one finger after the other, from the little finger to the thumb. Then, in a flowing movement, bend the wrists and elbows, too.

5, 6, and 7. Now push the arms gently to the sides to shoulder height, open the palms upwards, and roll the hands up once again.

8. Take the hands forward again and allow a very flowing and soft movement to occur. When breathing in, imagine gathering fresh energy via your hands and taking it all in. When breathing out, visualize that you are bringing used Chi out into your energy field where it can get neutralized.

Then take the hands onto your legs and feel the effect of the breath.

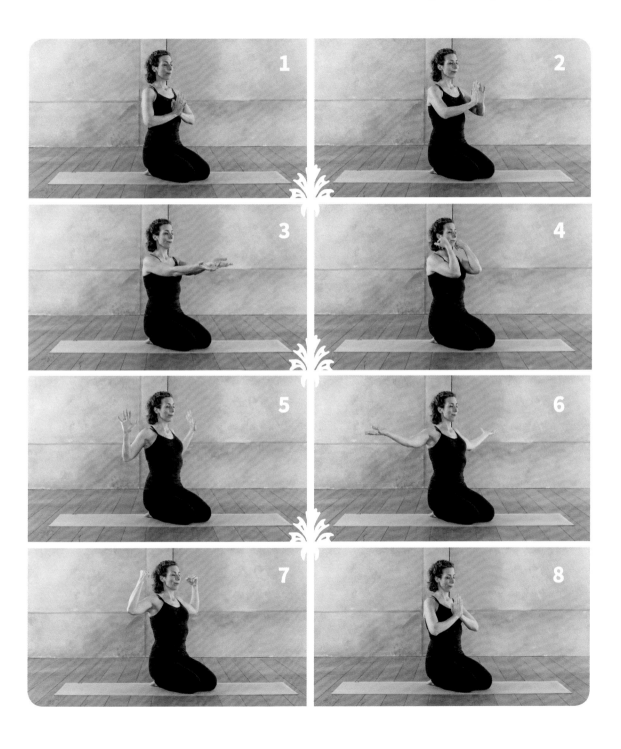

❀ Alternate Nostril Breathing

Alternate Nostril Breathing has a balancing effect, as you harmonize both of the main energy channels, Ida and Pingala, which correspond to Yin and Yang. Do Alternate Nostril Breathing until you feel balanced.

Practicing the exercise

Sit on the mat in Easy Pose and straighten your spine. Bend the index finder and middle finger of the right hand to the palm (the left-handed may wish to do the left), and stretch the ring finger and small finger out loosely. You can also place the index finger and middle finger on the third eye chakra (see page 27). Now close the left nostril with the ring finger and the right nostril with the thumb. Hold your nose very gently without applying any pressure. Keep your head straight and your right elbow to the side of your body. Start by inhaling on the left side, holding the right nostril closed while doing this. After inhaling, close the left side again, open the right, and take a long breath out. Then inhale again on the right and exhale again on the left. That is one complete breathing cycle.

You can also hold your breath between inhaling and exhaling. Ideally, the exhale should be longer than the inhale. (The two-eight-four rhythm is often recommended here for breathing in, holding, and breathing out, but this cycle can also be shortened or extended. Always adapt the breathing to your own requirements and capabilities.) Then let your hand sink down to your leg again and feel the effect.

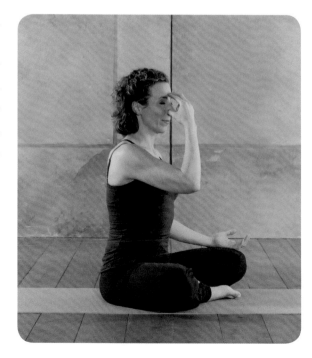

❀ Energy Breathing

This breathing technique has a very calming and harmonizing effect. You can do this either standing or sitting. Carry out as many cycles as you feel is right for you.

Practicing the exercise

1. Stand with legs hip-width apart and straighten your spine. Inhale, and raise your arms up sideways until your hands are touching above your head.

2. Exhale again, and take your hands above your heart to the center of energy underneath your navel. You can either place the hands over one another, or to the left and right of your navel. Pause for a moment before you start the next cycle. When inhaling, you can imagine collecting energy, and when you exhale, visualize how you are bringing the Chi energy to your center of energy.

Then remain standing with your hands on your stomach and feel the effect.

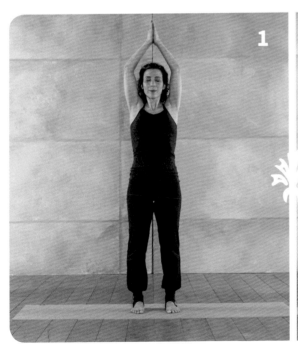 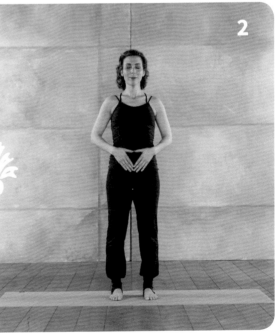

❦ Full Breathing

This breathing technique is very gentle and calming, and also good for beginners to do. Do Full Breathing as long as it feels comfortable.

Practicing the exercise

Sit on the mat in Easy Pose and straighten your spine. Be aware of your natural flow of breath. Let it deepen with every breath. Place your hands on your abdomen, left and right of your navel, and consciously direct your breath there. Then take the hands onto the lower ribcage and breathe into your chest area. Place your hands below your collarbone and breathe into the upper apex of the lungs. As you inhale, lift the hands upwards or forwards, and lower them again as you exhale. Put one hand on the lower abdomen and one hand on the upper abdomen. Now link up the breath across all three levels. Become aware of the small pauses between breathing in and out, and extend them a bit further. Now either breathe with an extended inhalation, very evenly, or with an extended exhalation—depending on what feels harmonious to you. However, always breathe in such a way that the breath can still flow easily.

Come back into the natural flow of breath and notice whether anything has changed.

Alternatively, you can also do Full Breathing while lying down. Place your feet on the floor and leave your hands resting on the abdomen. This version is ideal before going to sleep, for example, or if you are lying awake and unable to sleep at night.

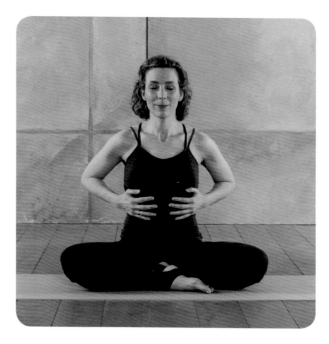

❀ Ujjayi Breathing

Ujjayi Breathing can create heat in the body, but it can also be very relaxing. It is therefore ideal for the start of practicing exercises, if you feel unsettled, or your mind is very full. Ujjayi translates as "victorious breathing," as it triumphs over shallow breathing. Breathe in Ujjayi as long as you like. In some styles of Yang Yoga, Ujjayi Breathing is also practiced while doing the poses.

Practicing the exercise

Sit in Easy Pose on the mat, and straighten your spine while placing your hands loosely on your legs. Now let the epiglottis narrow, with a deep flow of breath out into the throat area, as though you were making a whispering sound with your mouth closed or were breathing onto a mirror to clean it. The sound of Ujjayi Breathing is reminiscent of a distant sound of the sea. With this sound in the throat, you can inhale and exhale calmly and deeply.

Come back into a natural flow of breath and feel the effect.

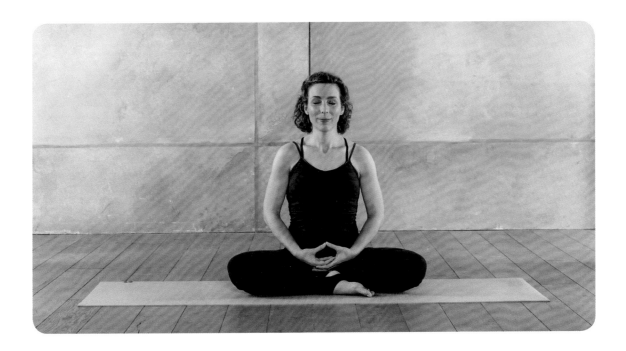

❀ The Healing **Meditations**

We live in a Yang-orientated world, in which there is often no place for stillness and inner contempla-tion. Most meditations have a Yin character and can therefore nicely balance out the overstimulation we feel every day. A demand for perfection is completely out of place here, and even if you only have time for a five-minute meditation each day, it can still have a great effect.

Breath Meditation

Breath Meditation is ideal for anyone who has not had any experience with meditation.

Practicing the exercise

You can practice breath meditation in Easy Pose, in the Ankle Stretch, or sitting comfortably on the mat with outstretched legs. If you wish, sit in a raised position, perhaps on a cushion or a meditation stool. If you have difficulties keeping your back straight, you can also lean against a wall. Now connect with your breath. Observe how your breath flows in and out naturally, and watch each individual breath. If you connect with your breath, then you are right in the present, as your breath always takes place in the now. Nevertheless, should you digress in your thoughts, then you can count your breaths. You either count each individual breath, or count the length in heartbeats or seconds. Identify for yourself when you would like to come out of your meditation, then slowly open your eyes and move your limbs.

Cleansing Meditation

Practice this meditation daily as you wish, as long as you feel completely freed by this.

Practicing the exercise

Recall something that made you feel uncomfortable: something that annoyed you, for example, or an injustice that was done to you or something that sucks your energy. Now think of an energizing place in nature, a place where you really feel good. Sense this place precisely. Imagine gentle drops of rain falling on you, which are colored violet. These drops are running over your whole body, first outside and then inside too—like an external and internal shower. The violet water flows over your hands and feet and out of you again, and takes everything with it that should no longer be part of you. If you feel externally and internally cleansed, then imagine your crown chakra (see page 27) opening up and radiant white light flowing into you. The rays are flowing through your whole body, and they replace everything that you have just given up with new positive energy and strength.

Protective Meditation

You can carry out this meditation any time you need protection on an energetic level.

Practicing the exercise

Concentrate on a color that gives you strength. Now imagine a column of light appearing in front of you in this color. Take a step forward in your mind and place yourself into the light. You are completely protected in this column of light. It connects you with the energy of the earth on the one hand, and with the energy of the sky on the other hand. You can help the effect further and use the following affirmation if it feels right to you: "May only light and loving energies come through to me, and may all negative energies remain outside, starting now." Then give thanks to the universe for this energetic protection.

Stillness Meditation

Stillness Meditation can be a challenge, but is also particularly inspiring.

Practicing the exercise

Go into Easy Pose. You can close your eyes or leave them open slightly. Now be aware of your body, and do not evaluate anything in doing so, but simply observe. How do you feel in your body today? Stay like this for a moment and direct your attention to your breath and your breathing. How is your breath flowing? Then direct your attention to your mind and observe its activity. How are you feeling at the moment on the mental level? Now, with each breath, let yourself go more and more, and allow yourself to be immersed in the inner stillness. If thoughts emerge, just take note of them and let them draw away again. Come back to stillness in yourself. You might take note of images here, or an inner voice, perhaps emotions, old memories, or experiences. Try not to assess anything, but just perceive it and what it is showing you. Let your meditation take place in stillness, without expecting anything. Stay in this as long as you wish. Then come back to yourself very gently. Feel your breath deepen, slowly open your eyes, and direct your gaze calmly to the floor once again. When you have finished, then ease out of your position.

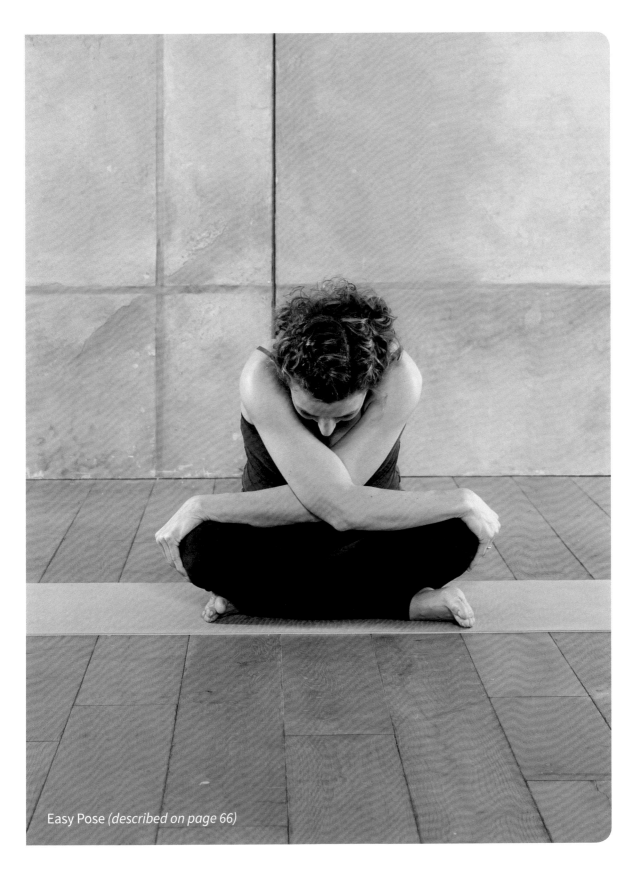

Easy Pose *(described on page 66)*

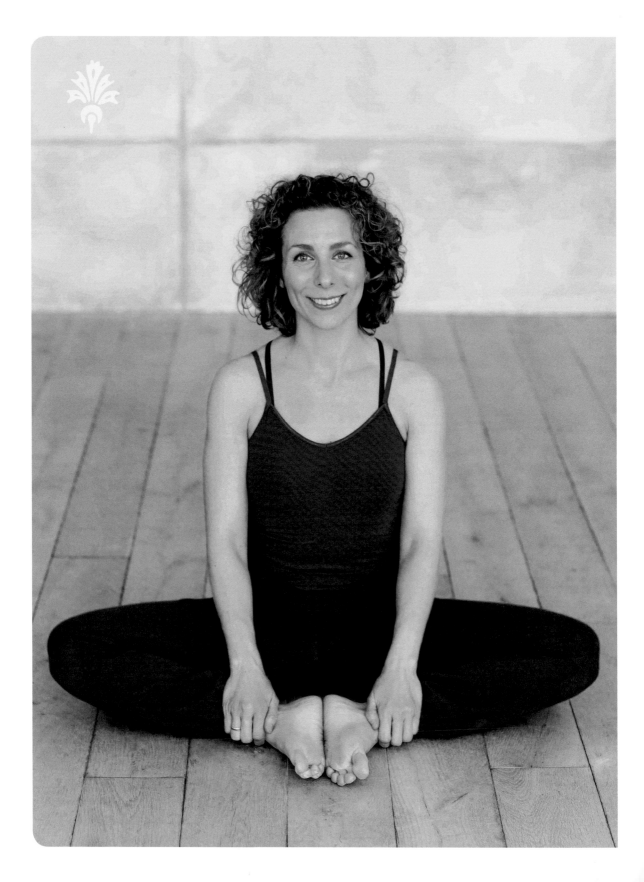

Yin Yoga for Health and Well-Being

Whether it is knee pain, anxiety, or skin problems, a targeted Yin Yoga practice offers gentle help with a variety of complaints. A Yin Yoga sequence has a very similar effect on our energies as an acupuncture treatment. The following sequences therefore correspond to the meridians that are relevant, from a TCM perspective, to the triggering of a healing process for a specific condition. You can therefore decide how long you hold the positions or how intensively you carry them out, on a completely individual basis and depending on how you feel each day.

❀ Agitation

The causes of general agitation are difficult to name. Agitation or nervousness is quite normal in some situations—in public appearances, before examinations, or before an important meeting with your boss, for example. Excessive consumption of caffeine, alcohol, or sugar can provoke restlessness. Sensitive people react to small amounts of these stimulants. However, general restlessness is often clearly a result of too much stress. If great responsibility falls upon your shoulders and your calender is permanently overfilled, it is difficult to switch off. Another disrupter of calm is the sensory overload to which we are all exposed nowadays; another is the presence of too much electronic smog in our close environment. Ultimately, certain illnesses can cause agitation—for example, heart problems, depression, or an overactive thyroid. A general agitation is also not uncommon during menopause.

From a holistic perspective, general agitation represents emotional imbalance. Your demands of yourself may be too high, and you may not have come to terms with yourself, or you may have lost contact with your internal center. Inner tension is possibly not recognized, and so cannot be processed and builds up into a blockage.

❀ **Possible questions for reflection are:**
What provides me with inner peace and calm?
What makes me nervous and how can I influence these factors?
What is missing to make me feel completely centered again?

In TCM, for agitation the liver, large intestine, heart, and kidneys are treated.

❀ If you often feel agitated, I recommend a daily meditation practice. Breathing exercises, in which you always consciously connect with your breath, are also beneficial. Your own breath can act like an inner anchor, even in situations that cause agitation, and this can bring you security and calmness. Yin Yoga practice provides wonderful peaceful energy, which can have a lasting effect if carried out with a certain degree of regularity. Sometimes, working out at a physical level can also help. Whether jogging in the fresh air, trampolining, or zumba, demanding sporting activities are ideal to quickly release excess tension. ❀

In addition to the **meridian massage** (page 36), I recommend this **Yin Yoga sequence:**

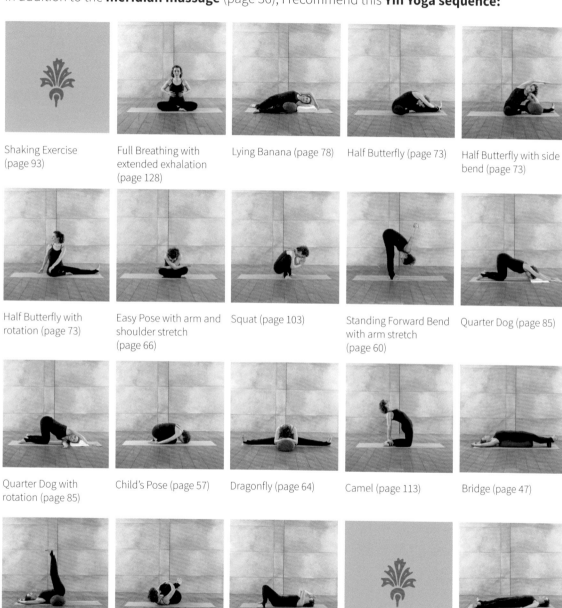

Shaking Exercise (page 93)

Full Breathing with extended exhalation (page 128)

Lying Banana (page 78)

Half Butterfly (page 73)

Half Butterfly with side bend (page 73)

Half Butterfly with rotation (page 73)

Easy Pose with arm and shoulder stretch (page 66)

Squat (page 103)

Standing Forward Bend with arm stretch (page 60)

Quarter Dog (page 85)

Quarter Dog with rotation (page 85)

Child's Pose (page 57)

Dragonfly (page 64)

Camel (page 113)

Bridge (page 47)

Seagrass (page 92)

Folded Pose (page 117)

Resting Pose (page 89)

Stillness Meditation (page 132)

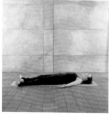

Relaxed Supine Position (page 87)

❧ **Allergies**

Living with an allergy always means restrictions for the person affected, as they constantly have to avoid potential allergens. Allergies often express themselves via the skin in the form of redness or rashes, as well as via the respiratory system or the mucous membranes. They provoke immune responses such as swellings, and are often accompanied by itchiness. There are many allergy triggers—pollen, for example, or grass, household dust, animal hairs, foods, cosmetics, or medicines. Why allergies are currently on the increase is not completely clear. It is assumed that environmental toxins—as well as a lack of contact with healthy germs, mostly in childhood—could be a possible cause.

From a holistic perspective, an allergy also has to do with rejection of a specific thing or person; for example, we might say "I have an allergic reaction to him or her" if we really do not like someone.

❧ **Possible questions for reflection are:**

To whom or what do I react, in my life or in myself, with rejection?
What topic have I not yet integrated into my life?
What upsets me and what do I react to? What am I intolerant of?
Where can I not yet set boundaries?

From the TCM perspective, allergies are about a weakness in the Chi of the immune system, which can be due to a lack of energy in the functional circuits of the lungs, spleen, and/or kidneys.

❧ With allergies it is advisable to consider treating the intestine, as it is largely responsible for our immune function. Those affected should have regular intestinal cleansing treatments—for example, by eating psyllium husks and bentonite or grounded flaxseed, or via enemas or colonic irrigation, in which the intestine is flushed out. At the same time, it is important to build up the flora of the intestine with probiotics to make the intestine stronger over the long term. In terms of food, the greatest allergy triggers are wheat, eggs, peanuts, nuts, milk products, soy, fish, and crustaceans, as well as flavor enhancers and colorants. ❧

In addition to the **meridian massage** (page 36), I recommend this **Yin Yoga sequence:**

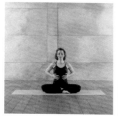

Full Breathing with extended exhalation (page 128)

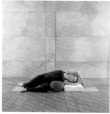

Lying Banana (page 78)

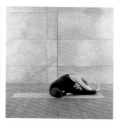

Half Butterfly (page 73)

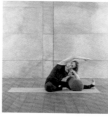

Half Butterfly with side bend (page 73)

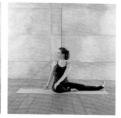

Half Butterfly with rotation (page 73)

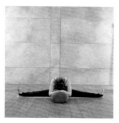

Dragonfly (page 64)

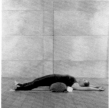

Rainbow Bridge (page 86)

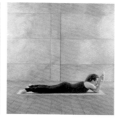

Sphinx with shoulder stretch (page 99)

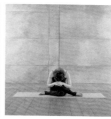

Shoelace (page 94)

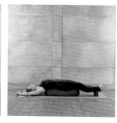

Bridge (page 47)

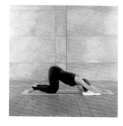

Quarter Dog (page 85)

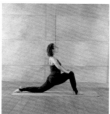

Dragon with intensified back bend (page 62)

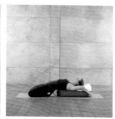

Downward Facing Dog (page 115)

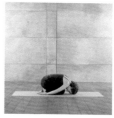

Saddle (page 90)

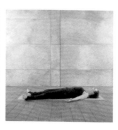

Child's Pose (page 57)

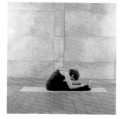

Caterpillar (page 51)

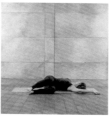

Twisted Roots (page 106)

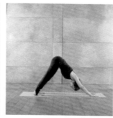

Resting Pose (page 89)

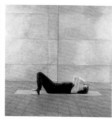

Breath Meditation (page 131)

Relaxed Supine Position (page 87)

❧ Anger and Teeth Grinding

Everyone knows emotions such as joy, sadness, anger, uncertainty, anxiety, or love. Children still live out their feelings in full. The older we become, the more we learn to manipulate our emotions—because in Western culture, unfortunately, they are categorized as good or bad. Illnesses may therefore arise at a deep level. Many people express suppressed emotions by grinding or pressing together their teeth, particularly when sleeping.

From a holistic perspective, emotions are neither positive nor negative, even if we are inclined to evaluate them this way. Emotions cannot be permanently suppressed or held under, and they persist until they are accepted. It is only then that they start to heal. As emotions are also anchored in the tissues of the body, they may come to the surface again through an intensive Yin Yoga practice. If that is the case, a valuable cleansing process takes place, which encourages acceptance and letting go.

❧ Possible questions for reflection are:

Am I allowed to live out my emotions, or do I suppress them?
How can I resolve my pattern of thinking that emotions are good or bad?
What is it inside me that wants to be seen or gain more attention?

From a TCM perspective, anger and fury belong to the liver and gallbladder functional circuit. This may also have to do with long-suppressed emotions or even issues from childhood; it does not have to be a current situation.

> ❧ If you see yourself confronted with emotions that you would rather suppress, then please try this little meditation. Sit up straight or lie down. Recall an unpleasant feeling—anger, annoyance, anxiety, sadness, or whatever comes to mind. Name this feeling and welcome it. Meet your emotions and feel them openly without rejecting them. Also ask yourself why they are there and what they want to show you. Watch how your emotions change the more you watch them mindfully. Perhaps they become less intense and seem a little less threatening. If you accept your feelings, you can also let go of them more easily via the process of accepting them. ❧

In addition to the **meridian massage** (page 36), I recommend this **Yin Yoga sequence:**

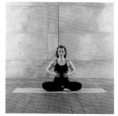

Full Breathing with extended breathing (page 128)

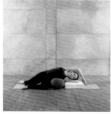

Lying Banana (page 78)

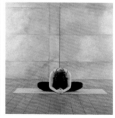

Butterfly (page 48)

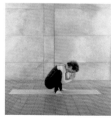

Squat (page 103)

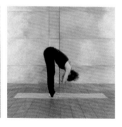

Standing Forward Bend (page 60)

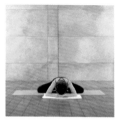

Frog (page 71)

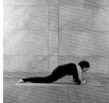

Dragon (page 62)

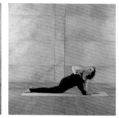

Dragon with rotation (page 62)

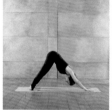

Downward Facing Dog (page 115)

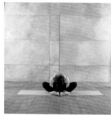

Turtle (page 104)

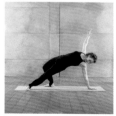

Tripod (page 122)

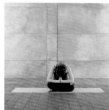

Square (page 101)

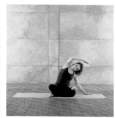

Square with side bend (page 101)

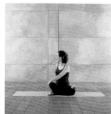

Square with rotation (page 101)

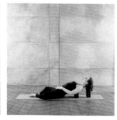

Lying Butterfly (page 79)

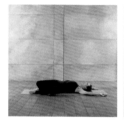

Dynamic Windshield Wiper (page 116)

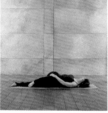

Twisted roots with intensified rotation (page 106)

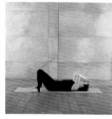

Resting Pose (page 89)

Stillness Meditation page 132)

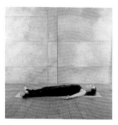

Relaxed Supine Position (page 87)

✺ Anxieties

There are many kinds of anxieties, and most are associated with loss of confidence—particularly our basic trust, which is marked in childhood. Anxiety is often noticeable at the physical level—for example, through increased blood pressure, tense muscles, and especially in the breathing. With anxiety states, the breathing becomes quick and flat, and there is often a feeling of narrowing or rigidity. Besides this, anxiety has an important protective effect, as it makes us attentive to real situations of danger.

From a holistic perspective, it is important to face your fear in order to find out its cause. Anyone confronted by anxieties should go through them and not run away from them. (This does not apply to traumatized or depressed people, who should always work with a therapist and not face these issues alone.) A state of anxiety often resolves itself quickly if you stand up to it, like a dark cloud passing. What is important is to strengthen the basic trust again, and constantly ground yourself—for example, by walking in the countryside, frequently sitting on the ground, walking barefoot, or working in the garden. Depending on how deep the anxieties are, working with a therapist can be very helpful. In China there is a lovely expression which goes: "Anxiety knocked on the door, trust opened it, and nobody was there."

✺ **Possible questions for reflection are:**

What exactly do I fear?
What is the trigger for my anxiety?
Where and how can I feel this anxiety?
What happens when I face the anxiety?
What happens if I feed my anxiety with trust and love?

✺ For anxieites I recommend a vegetarian diet, as meat can be negatively charged from a spiritual perspective. Anxieties that the slaughtered animal experienced just before death can still be stored in the meat at an energetic level, and can be transferred to the person eating it. Besides giving up meat products (the same can apply to fish), adding grounding foods to the diet can have a balancing effect and give energy. Potatoes and root vegetables—carrots, for example, and beetroot, parsnips, and celeriac—should be on the shopping list as often as possible. ✺

From the TCM perspective, there are many causes of anxiety, many of which are treated differently. You often hear of a disharmony between the heart and kidneys, but the spleen, liver, and large intestine may also play a part here.

In addition to the **meridian massage** (page 36), I recommend this **Yin Yoga sequence:**

Shaking Exercise (page 93)

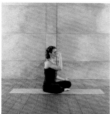

Alternate Nostril Breathing (page 126)

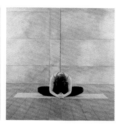

Butterfly (page 48)

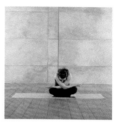

Easy Pose with arm and shoulder stretch (page 66)

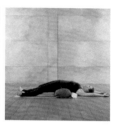

Rainbow Bridge (page 86)

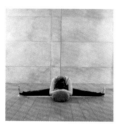

Dragonfly (page 64)

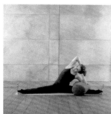

Dragonfly with side bend (page 64)

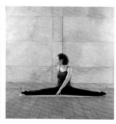

Dragonfly with rotation (page 64)

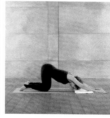

Quarter Dog (page 85)

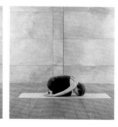

Child's Pose (page 57)

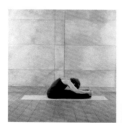

Caterpillar with acupressure point bubbling spring (page 51)

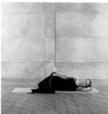

Cat Pulling Its Tail (page 50)

Meridian Tapping Massage (page 41)

Protective Meditation (page 132)

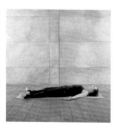

Relaxed Supine Position (page 87)

❀ Arthrosis

Arthrosis is caused by wear and tear of the joint cartilage, which causes tension, swelling, deformities, stiffness, inflammation, and pains in the joint. Almost all joints can be affected by arthrosis, but it is particularly common in the knee and hip joints.

From a holistic perspective, arthrosis can be an indication of a way of thinking that is too rigid. It is possible you do not move as freely in life as you did in your younger years. Introspection through regular meditation, for example, can therefore be all the more important.

❀ **Possible questions for reflection are:**
Whereabouts do I feel restricted in my life?
Where have I become rigid in my habits, and where can I be more flexible?

In TCM, the lungs and spleen are taken into consideration when treating arthrosis. Other important factors are the meridians where complaints show up, in particular:
- **Jaw:** stomach, triple warmer, large intestine, and possibly the small intestine (depending on the location)
- **Shoulders:** triple warmer, large intestine, small intestine, gallbladder, and stomach
- **Cervical spine:** gallbladder, bladder, small intestine, and possibly the triple warmer
- **Elbows, hands, and fingers:** triple warmer, small intestine, and large intestine
- **Thoracic spine:** bladder and small intestine
- **Lumbar spine:** governing vessel, bladder, and (if feeling cold) kidney
- **Sacroiliac joint:** bladder and kidney
- **Hips:** gallbladder (as the most important meridian) and bladder
- **Knees:** kidney, stomach, gallbladder, liver, and spleen
- **Feet:** gallbladder, stomach, bladder, spleen, liver, kidney, and large intestine
- **Toes:** spleen, stomach, kidney, bladder, gallbladder, and large intestine

> ❀ With arthrosis, it is important to reduce excess body weight, limit inflammatory reactions, and improve the metabolic process in the joint. Alkaline nutrition that is rich in minerals and trace elements can be of help here. Omega-3–rich vegetable fats, fruit, vegetables, and whole-grain products should often be in the diet (no wheat if you are gluten-sensitive); meat, eggs, caffeine, alcohol, too much sugar, and processed products should be consumed as little as possble. Perfect thirst-quenchers are non-carbonated water and herbal teas. ❀

In addition to the **meridian massage** (page 36), I recommend this **Yin Yoga sequence:**

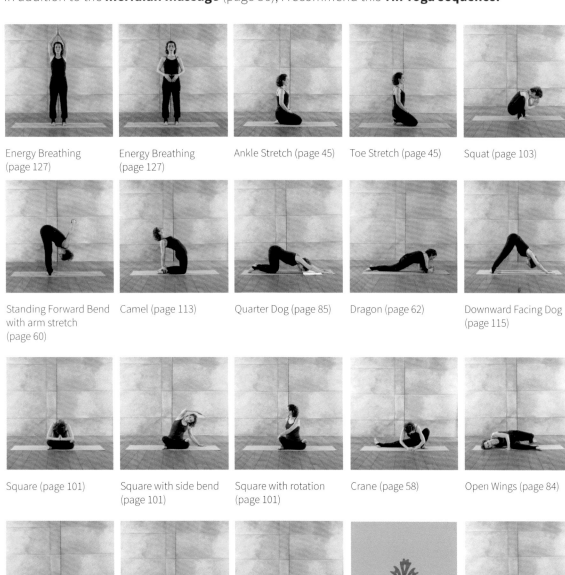

Energy Breathing
(page 127)

Energy Breathing
(page 127)

Ankle Stretch (page 45)

Toe Stretch (page 45)

Squat (page 103)

Standing Forward Bend
with arm stretch
(page 60)

Camel (page 113)

Quarter Dog (page 85)

Dragon (page 62)

Downward Facing Dog
(page 115)

Square (page 101)

Square with side bend
(page 101)

Square with rotation
(page 101)

Crane (page 58)

Open Wings (page 84)

Embracing Wings
(page 67)

Saddle (page 90)

Twisted Roots with
intensified stretch
(page 106)

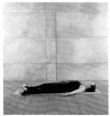

Stillness Meditation
(page 132)

Relaxed Supine Position
(page 87)

❧ Bladder Complaints

Women in particular often suffer from bladder complaints. Most will experience a bladder infection once in their life, and many will experience it several times. Possible causes of these complaints include hypothermia, scar tissue in the abdomen, repeatedly holding urine, weak pelvic floor muscles, sexual activity, clothing that is too tight and doesn't "breathe," and poor posture.

From a holistic perspective, bladder complaints are associated with the themes of accumulating, withstanding, and letting go. It is therefore about letting go of what has outlived its purpose, instead of holding onto it. Those who suffer frequently from bladder infections are often under too much pressure and tension. There can be a direct link to the sacral chakra (see page 27).

❧ **Possible questions for reflection are:**
Am I under negative pressure? If so, what can I do about it?
Why is it so difficult for me to let go, and how can I do it better?
How can I better enter into the flow of life again?

From a TCM perspective, in the case of frequently recurring bladder complaints, the functional circuit of the kidneys and bladder should be treated. It is also important to identify the type and cause of the complaint: if it is a bacterial bladder infection, then the spleen and stomach are the basis (nourishing energy) of the defense Chi; the lungs should also be taken into account for their defense energy. However, if it is an irritable bladder, then it is likely that you will have to look to the functional circuit of the heart / small intestine instead.

> ❧ When bladder infections occur frequently, cranberry juice has proven to be the best remedy; ¼ to ½ liter per day can prevent urinary infections. Cranberries contain a flavonoid that stops the bacteria adhering to the wall of the bladder. The antioxidants in blueberries, celery, carrots, papaya, and parsley promote the health of the bladder. Celery has pain-limiting, infection-inhibiting, and diuretic properties. Parsley and carrots increase the flow of urine and strengthen the urinary tract. Blueberries have similar content to cranberries, and papaya can be a diuretic. With bladder infections, you should also drink a lot of water or bladder tea, and avoid irritants such as alcohol or caffeine. ❧

In addition to the **meridian massage** (page 36), I recommend this **Yin Yoga sequence:**

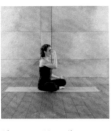

Alternate Nostril
Breathing (page 126)

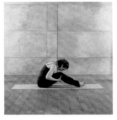

Coachman with
acupressure point
(page 51)

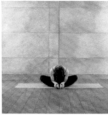

Turtle with acupressure
point (page 104)

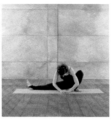

Crane (page 58)

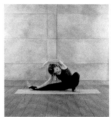

Crane with side bend
(page 58)

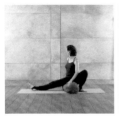

Crane with rotation
(page 58)

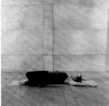

Dynamic Windshield
Wiper (page 116)

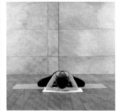

Frog (page 71)

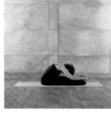

Caterpillar with
acupressure point
bubbling spring
(page 51)

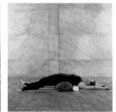

Rainbow Bridge
(page 86)

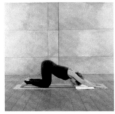

Quarter Dog (page 85)

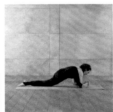

Dragon (page 62)

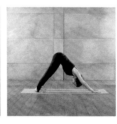

Downward Facing Dog
(page 115)

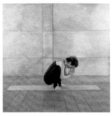

Squat (page 103)

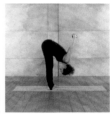

Standing Forward Bend
with arm stretch
(page 60)

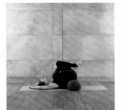

Eye of the Needle
(page 68)

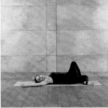

Eye of the Needle with
rotation (page 68)

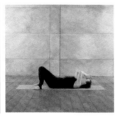

Resting Pose (page 89)

Stillness Meditation
(page 132)

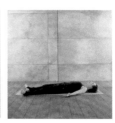

Relaxed Supine Position
(page 87)

❦ Burnout Syndrome

Burnout syndrome is a state of total exhaustion, which may be physical, emotional, or mental, or a combination of all of them. Never have so many people been burnt out as in recent times, which can certainly be attributed to a lifestyle that has too much Yang energy and is characterized by constant accessibility and an ever-increasing pressure to perform. Burnout is frequently the precursor to depression, and does not come about overnight. For this reason, it is important to factor in short rest periods in stressful everyday life. Even a small break of two minutes, in which the focus is placed consciously on the breathing, can charge the whole system and bring new energy. Excessive media consumption is a real energy-sapper. TVs, smartphones, and computers do not belong in the bedroom and should be switched off at night—this should be obvious.

From a holistic perspective, energy reserves are completely exhausted in those affected by burnout, and even a short-term recovery does not help. It is therefore important to interpret these clear signals from the body: in order to gain space for personal introspection, treat yourself to extended periods of rest, allow yourself to get enough sleep, keep some distance from stressful everyday life, and practice conscious withdrawal. Yoga and meditation can be very helpful in this way.

❀ **Possible questions for reflection are:**

Who or what in my life is depleting my energy?

What are my inner resources and sources of energy?

How can I defend myself better against negative stress?

What tasks can I delegate to have more time to myself?

❀ As food can be a giver of energy as well as a taker, those suffering from burnout should take care with their diet. A natural diet, with a high proportion of fresh fruit and vegetables, salads, nuts, seeds, herbs, wild herbs, spices, whole-grain products, healthy fats, and a lot of (non-carbonated) water as a main drink, can have a balancing and strengthening effect. Smoothies or fresh juices can also quickly supply energy. Fast foods and stimulants such as caffeine, sugar, tobacco, and nicotine only give a good feeling in the short term, but viewed over the long term they actually also pollute the body. ❀

From the TCM perspective, this has to do with a disharmony between the heart and kidney. The liver and large intestine should be decongested. The following should also be treated:

- For heart-circulation problems: heart, small intestine, and bladder
- For stomach-intestine-problems: spleen, stomach, and lungs
- For weak muscles: spleen
- For a weak spine: governing vessel
- For a weak immune system: lungs

In addition to the **meridian massage** (page 36), I recommend this **Yin Yoga sequence:**

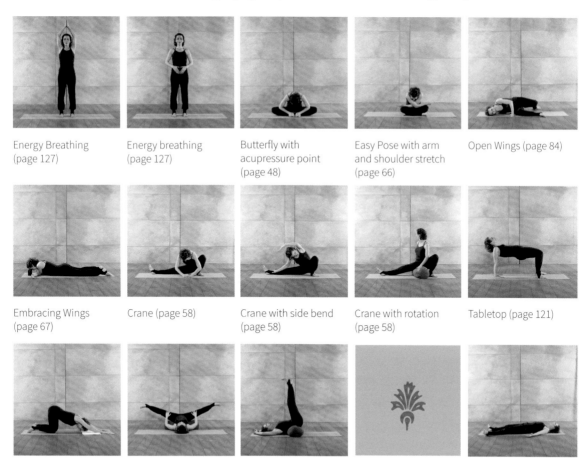

Energy Breathing (page 127)

Energy breathing (page 127)

Butterfly with acupressure point (page 48)

Easy Pose with arm and shoulder stretch (page 66)

Open Wings (page 84)

Embracing Wings (page 67)

Crane (page 58)

Crane with side bend (page 58)

Crane with rotation (page 58)

Tabletop (page 121)

Quarter Dog (page 85)

Dragonfly in back position (page 64)

Seagrass (page 92)

Stillness Meditation (page 132)

Relaxed Supine Position (page 87)

⚜ Cellulite

Cellulite has to do with a change in the subcutaneous tissue; it manifests itself in dimpled skin and mainly appears on the upper thighs, buttocks, stomach, and upper arms. From a medical perspective it is not dangerous, but many dislike it for aesthetic reasons. Almost 80 percent of all women are affected by cellulite, as women have thinner skin and weaker connective tissue than men. The connective tissue of women also has to stretch sufficiently in pregnancy, and therefore has a columnar structure. With men, the collagen and elastic fibers are arranged in a grid-like way so that it is not easy for cellulite to spread.

From a holistic perspective, weak connective tissue can be attributed to being too compliant (women often find it difficult to say no) or a lack of stability in your own life.

⚜ Possible questions for reflection are:

What gives me inner support?
What do I have to do to be able to say no?
How can I ensure I have boundaries?
What do I need to feel stable in my life?

From a TCM perspective, it is the spleen that is treated for weaknesses of the connective tissue. The spleen is responsible for the connective tissue and support function: it holds the blood in the vessels (where there is a weakness of the spleen, there is a tendency towards bruising) and keeps the internal organs in place.

⚜ Yin Yoga can be excellent for fighting cellulite, as the deep stretches of fascia stimulate the flow of lymph. You can also work with foam rollers or fascia balls to roll out the whole body, particularly at the weak points where cellulite shows. Two to three sessions per week are sufficient. Fantastic results can also be obtained from cupping therapy: this allows a vacuum to emerge in the connective tissue, which helps to remove old low-nutrient tissue water and exchanges it for fresh supplies that have dense nutrients. If you are looking for anti-cellulite training with a great deal of power and which is plenty of fun, you should try out trampolining. ⚜

In addition to the **meridian massage** (page 36), I recommend this **Yin Yoga sequence:**

Shaking Exercise
(page 93)

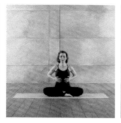
Full Breathing with
extended exhalation
(page 128)

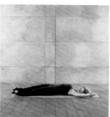
Lying Half Moon
(page 80)

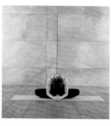
Butterfly (page 48)

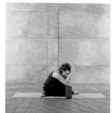
Shoelace shoulder
stretch (page 94)

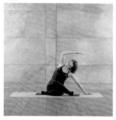
Shoelace with side bend
(page 94)

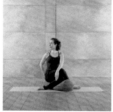
Shoelace with rotation
(page 94)

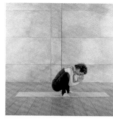
Squat (page 103)

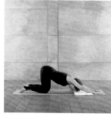
Quarter Dog (page 85)

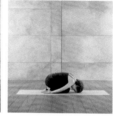
Child's Pose (page 57)

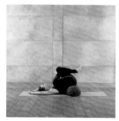
Eye of the Needle
(page 68)

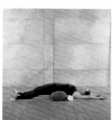
Rainbow Bridge
(page 86)

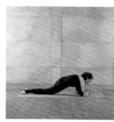
Dragon (page 62)

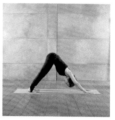
Downward Facing Dog
(page 115)

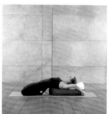
Saddle (page 90)

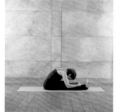
Caterpillar (page 51)

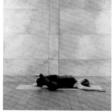
Twisted Roots with
intensified stretch
(page 106)

Meridian Tapping
Massage (page 41)

Protective Meditation
(page 132)

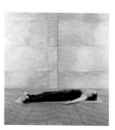
Relaxed Supine Position
(page 87)

❦ Complaints During Pregnancy

Pregnancy is an intensive time, where it is important to care for yourself and the growing baby lovingly. As the body of the expectant mother is having to perform in a truly unbelievable way, the pregnant mother should make it a priority to be able to say no—especially when it comes to things and people that sap the energy. This has a direct effect on the baby, as well as on the birth. I had no experience of yoga at the time of my first pregnancy and was caught up in Yang energy, only taking very little time for myself. This was reflected in the pregnancy as well as the birth. I went into labor very early (18 weeks), and had to take a tocolytic to not lose my baby; the birth extended over 39 hours. With the second pregnancy, when I was already familiar with yoga, everything went very differently. Although my body reacted with early labor once again, I was able to counter it through my yoga practice and did not need any medicines. It was also a very pleasant birth that only took a few hours. Many of the pregnant participants in my yoga classes told me later that their babies were very balanced and did not cry much. As Yin Yoga tends to emphasize our feminine side, it is ideally suited for this time in a woman's life. If you follow a few key principles, there is nothing to recommend against a regular Yin Yoga practice during pregnancy.

Pregnant women should always stretch gently and not include the stomach area too intensively; props such as yoga bolsters, blankets, and cushions can help with this. During pregnancy, the hormone relaxin also ensures that women's bodies become increasingly softer, so that the muscle

❋ Nutrition plays a particularly important role for the expectant mother. The idea of having to eat for two relates less to the size of the portions, however, and much more to the content of the food. During pregnancy, the body runs at full speed and requires adequate high-quality nutrients to supply the mother and baby with sufficient energy. Of particular significance are iron, iodine, and folic acid, which are to be found in amaranth, quinoa, pumpernickel, oats, millet, dates, dried apricots and figs (non-sulphurized), sesame, nuts, seaweed, green leafy vegetables, broccoli, wild herbs, basil, parsley, raisins, bananas, oranges, dark berries, yeast flakes, beetroot, potatoes, and legumes. As pregnant women react more sensitively, the well-known sudden cravings often give an indication of whether the body is lacking a specific nutrient. ❋

tone is reduced somewhat and the ligaments yield. Therefore, many women are more mobile during pregnancy than they were before. However, there is still a risk of injury if stretches are carried out too intensely. You should also monitor the length of time for holding individual positions, as a shorter time is usually more appropriate.

Care should also be taken with rotations, as this should only be done on the open side or in the thoracic spine. It is also recommended not to lie on your back for a long time, as the belly becomes larger with the progression of the pregnancy and the weight is therefore too heavy. Lying on your back may then cause too much pressure on the vena cava, which carries the blood to the heart. It is often more comfortable to lie on the left side. However, there is no general rule for everyone. When you are pregnant, you should simply observe your attention—as you feel it internally, at all times—to check which positions feel right and which do not. Always pay full heed to your inner yoga teacher and respect the signals from your body. If it feels good to you, then it is probably also doing your baby good.

During pregnancy, complaints such as sickness, major tiredness, and excessive weight gain or pregnancy diabetes may occur. In most cases, the adapting hormones are the reason for possible changes.

From a holistic perspective, an expectant mother should also be aware of the changes in life that she will encounter, and ask herself whether she has already accepted them internally or is still rebelling against them in the form of physical symptoms.

❧ **Possible questions for reflection are:**
Am I ready for my new role as mother, and how is my relationship with the father of the child?
What would I like to do differently from my own parents?
What aspects still remain to be healed in my relationship with my mother?

During pregnancy, **TCM** particularly treats the kidney, heart, and uterus, as well as the connections to the eight extraordinary vessels (see page 26), the liver, stomach, and spleen. The kidney stores the prenatal essence, and supplies the material basis for forming and maturing the nuclei and the formation of the menstrual blood. Along with the heart, it controls the beginning, the process, and the end of fertility. The heart houses the spirit ("Shen" in Chinese), and controls the eight extraordinary vessels and the circulation of the blood. It promotes ovulation, as well as the later expulsion of menstrual blood. The uterus regulates conception, pregnancy, birth, and menstruation, together with the ovaries, the fallopian tubes, and the uterine cervix.

The following **Yin Yoga sequence** is an option for addressing these meridians. However, you should decide for yourself, and vary it if some positions do not feel right.

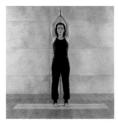

Energy Breathing (page 127)

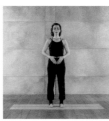

Energy Breathing (page 127)

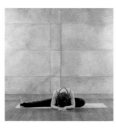

Half Dragonfly (page 64)

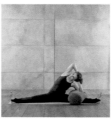

Dragonfly with side bend (page 64)

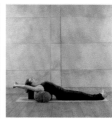

Fish (page 70)

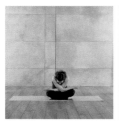

Easy Pose with arm and shoulder stretch (page 66)

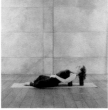

Lying Butterfly (page 79)

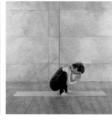

Squat (page 103)

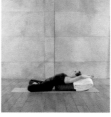

Half Lying Lotus (page 75)

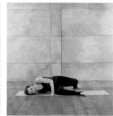

Open Wings (page 84)

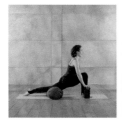

Dragon with blocks and yoga bolster (page 62)

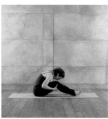

Coachman (page 51)

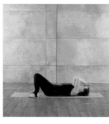

Resting Pose (page 89)

Breath Meditation (page 131)

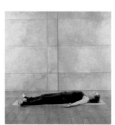

Relaxed Supine Position or on the side (page 87)

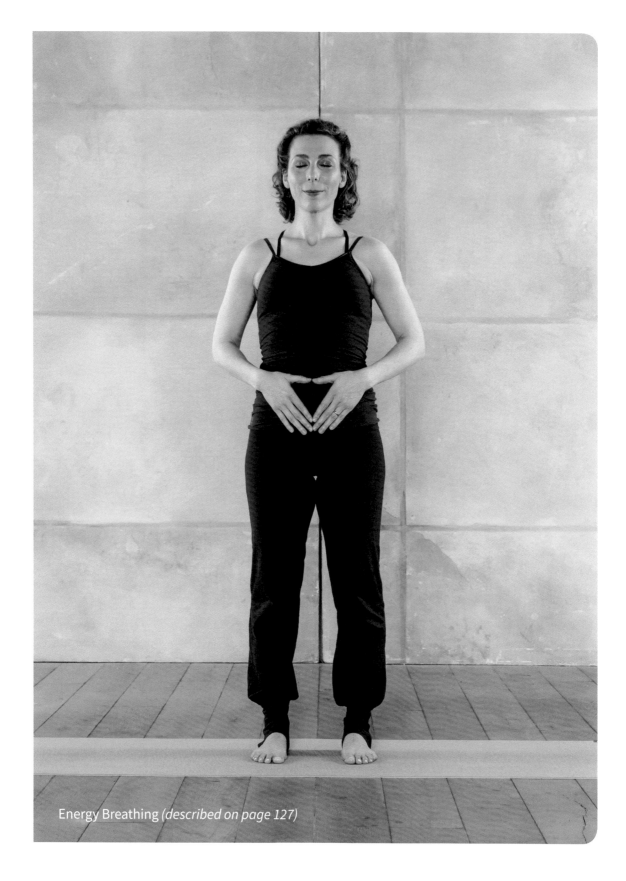

Energy Breathing (*described on page 127*)

❀ Depression

Depression is a psychological condition that is often accompanied by listlessness, tiredness, sadness, anxieties, feelings of guilt, and loss of performance, self-worth, or joy. It can have endogenous causes, but could also be of a psychogenic nature, i.e. related to conflicts, stressful circumstances, or trauma. Depression is oftentimes kept secret by its sufferers, due to embarrassment. If it is not just a temporary, slightly more depressive mood, but manifest depression, treatment via a psychotherapist is indicated. Yoga teachers should never presume to see themselves in this position without training in this field. However, they can give valuable support on the way to treatment and accompany the person affected on their journey.

From a holistic perspective, it is assumed that depression has to do with suppressed emotions—for example, with aggression, grief, or anger. It is therefore important to set out self-determined boundaries, and work through possible trauma or face your own anxieties. Meditation can be very helpful here, but the inexperienced should practice with a teacher who can help and support them if necessary.

❀ Possible questions for reflection are:

Why am I anxious?
Which of my emotions and experiences wish to be seen?
What issues from my childhood still need to be healed?
What is my calling, and how do I get back on my path?

From a TCM perspective, there are around twenty different types of depression with different patterns. A liver Chi stagnation is always treated for this, along with the large intestine; for deep brooding the spleen should be addressed as well, and for grief, the lungs.

> ❀ Depressive upsets can often be attributed to a lack of serotonin. This good mood hormone not only ensures greater calmness and a positive mood, but also reduces negative feelings and anxieties. A good opportunity to stimulate serotonin production is sports training—ideally in the daylight and sunshine, as light encourages the formation of the happiness hormone. ❀

In addition to the **meridian massage** (page 36), I recommend this **Yin Yoga sequence:**

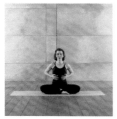

Full Breathing with extended exhalation (page 131)

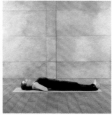

Twisted Arms (page 105)

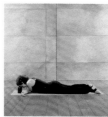

Rainbow Bridge (page 86)

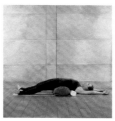

Embracing Wings (page 67)

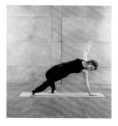

Tripod (page 122)

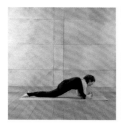

Dragon (page 62)

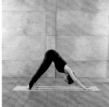

Downward Facing Dog (page 115)

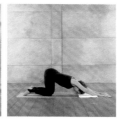

Quarter Dog (page 85)

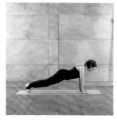

Plank (page 120)

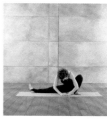

Crane (page 58)

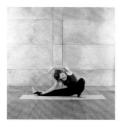

Crane with side bend (page 58)

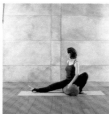

Crane with rotation (page 58)

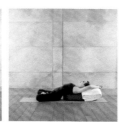

Half Lying Lotus (page 75)

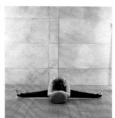

Dragonfly (page 64)

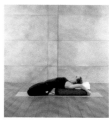

Saddle (page 90)

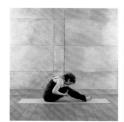

Coachman (page 51)

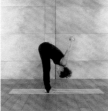

Standing Forward Bend with arm stretch (page 60)

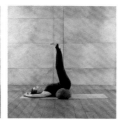

Seagrass (page 92)

Cleansing Meditation (page 131)

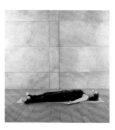

Relaxed Supine Position (page 87)

❧ Digestive Complaints

There are many digestive complaints, but most have to do with heartburn, flatulence, diarrhea, or constipation. Those affected can do a lot to help themselves; whether it is sport, fitness exercises at work, or consistently climbing stairs, staying active stimulates the intestinal function. Our toilet habits also play a role. The most natural posture for evacuation is squatting. The toilets we use are built for sitting and do not allow this, and digestive complaints are therefore on the increase. One reason for this is that we can not evacuate a stool completely in the sitting position, as part of the intestine bends and the intestinal passage is impeded. A simple solution is offered by a standard stepstool, which you place in front of the toilet so that the feet are higher.

From a holistic perspective, digestive complaints are associated with impressions we are unable to process. It has often to do with the topic of letting go.

❧ Possible questions for reflection are:
What issues have I not yet digested?
What things are lying heavy with me?
What do I have to let go to free myself?

From a TCM perspective, there are many patterns of fullness and emptiness that can be attributed to various illnesses; essentially, any meridian may play a part here. In any case, stomach massage is recommended.

> ❧ Dietary fiber supports intestinal functioning, and this is contained particularly in fruit, salad, vegetables, whole-grain products, legumes, nuts, and seeds. What is important here is to drink a lot of water. Flatulance is often caused by cabbage and legumes, and some people also react to a surfeit of fiber. You have to listen to your own body here. This can be relieved by coriander, aniseed, fennel, and caraway. A true all-rounder is psyllium husks, a purely natural product that helps with both diarrhea and constipation. Besides this, psyllium husks can absorb toxins from the intestine and help excrete them. If you suffer frequently from heartburn, you should cut out sweet things, white flour products, alcohol, nicotine, coffee, fizzy sodas, tomatoes, hot spices, juice, and very salty or fatty foods. ❧

For digestive complaints I recommend a balanced **Yin Yoga sequence**, which addresses all meridians and moves the abdomen in all directions.

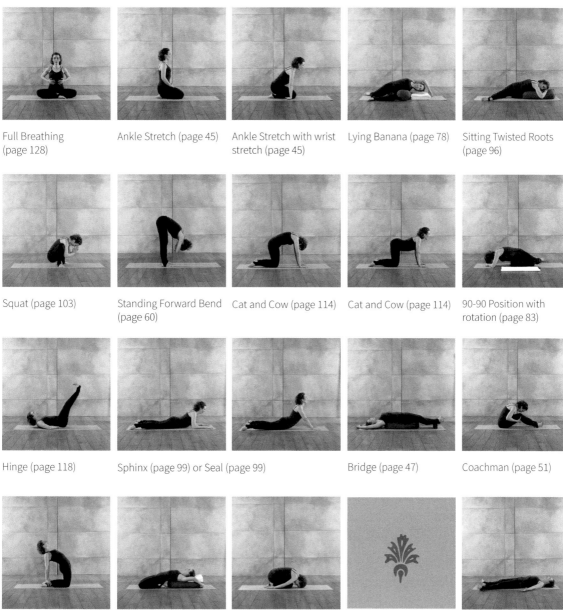

Full Breathing (page 128)

Ankle Stretch (page 45)

Ankle Stretch with wrist stretch (page 45)

Lying Banana (page 78)

Sitting Twisted Roots (page 96)

Squat (page 103)

Standing Forward Bend (page 60)

Cat and Cow (page 114)

Cat and Cow (page 114)

90-90 Position with rotation (page 83)

Hinge (page 118)

Sphinx (page 99) or Seal (page 99)

Bridge (page 47)

Coachman (page 51)

Camel (page 113)

Saddle (page 90)

Child's Pose (page 57)

Breath Meditation (page 131)

Relaxed Supine Position (page 87)

❋ Ear Problems

Our ears are not only sense organs; inside them is also the organ of balance that is so vital for us. The ears are very sensitive for many people, and they quickly react to drafts or water in the ear canal. Cold complaints are often also accompanied by an unpleasant stinging or pulling in the areas of the ears. Classic ear infections are usually very painful. Increasingly, people also suffer from tinnitus—a whistling, squeaking, or humming ear noise, which may be with the person affected day and night and can be very distressing. Not least, noise and loud music can stress our ears, so that major damage is a concern—especially among young people, who regularly wear earphones when on the move.

From a holistic perspective, the ears have to do with the notion of being obedient. Parents often say to their children that they must listen to what they say. This pattern continues throughout life: the student has to listen to the teacher, the employee has to listen to what the boss is dictating to them . . . If sufficient aggression and suppressed anger have built up, we might say that "we can't listen to another word of it."

❋ **Possible questions for reflection are:**
What do I not want to hear?
Do I have good contact with my inner voice?
Am I leading a self-determining life?

In TCM, it is assumed that the functioning of the kidney is weakened when hearing diminishes. It is a typical complaint of aging, which is based on the loss of energy in the kidneys. With repeated ear problems, you can strengthen the immune system by treating the lungs, triple warmer, spleen, stomach, large intestine, and gallbladder.

> ❋ **If pains keep occurring in the ears, you should check by temporarily cutting out the classic allergenic foods such as wheat, eggs, nuts, dairy products, additives such as glutamates, fish, crustaceans, or soy to see if the situation improves. With allergies, mucus is often produced, which collects in the nasal cavity and throat area and exerts painful pressure on the ears. An allergic reaction may also cause an ear infection.** ❋

In addition to the **meridian massage** (page 36), I recommend this **Yin Yoga sequence:**

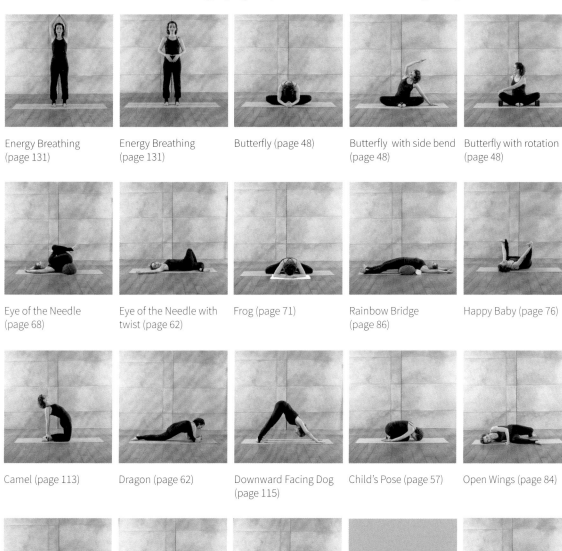

Energy Breathing
(page 131)

Energy Breathing
(page 131)

Butterfly (page 48)

Butterfly with side bend
(page 48)

Butterfly with rotation
(page 48)

Eye of the Needle
(page 68)

Eye of the Needle with
twist (page 62)

Frog (page 71)

Rainbow Bridge
(page 86)

Happy Baby (page 76)

Camel (page 113)

Dragon (page 62)

Downward Facing Dog
(page 115)

Child's Pose (page 57)

Open Wings (page 84)

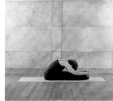

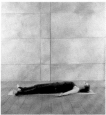

Embracing Wings
(page 67)

Cat Pulling Its Tail
(page 50)

Caterpillar with
acupressure point
(page 51)

Stillness Meditation
(page 132)

Relaxed Supine Position
(page 87)

❧ Eyesight Issues

Our eyes are called upon every day, and most people's eyesight declines during their lifetime. Smartphones and hours of work on the screen also stress the eyes. When the eyesight is deteriorating, however, there are things you can do to stabilize or even improve it again—for example, with classic eye yoga or targeted Yin Yoga sequences. All you need is consistency and some patience until the first signs of success become apparent.

From a holistic perspective, the eyes are the window of the soul. You can read from their eyes whether somebody is cheerful, sad, happy, angry, or worried. We first make contact with another person via the eyes. We look away if we do not want to have anything to do with a person or a thing.

❧ **Possible questions for reflection are:**
Who or what in my life do I not want to see?
How can I turn my gaze inwards better?
On what do I need to focus more in my life?

From the TCM perspective, the functioning of the liver and gallbladder are most important for the eyesight. You can also strengthen them if you include the center with the stomach and spleen.

❧ **If practiced each day, the following eye exercise can improve your eyesight. With your eyes open, move them side to side four to eight times, and then up and down, then diagonally from upper right to lower left, and then from upper left to lower right. Circle the eyes with a wide radius in both directions, and then do large figure eights. Then look closely and in the distance a few times—for example, at the tip of your nose and then through a window. Then close your eyes, let them rest and relax. This exercise can be rather unpleasant to start with, and in some cases it may cause slight nausea or faintness. That is usually a sign of strain. But do not be discouraged if this happens; just practice in small steps—gently—in order to strengthen your eye muscles over the long term. ❧**

In addition to the **meridian massage** (page 36), I recommend this **Yin Yoga sequence:**

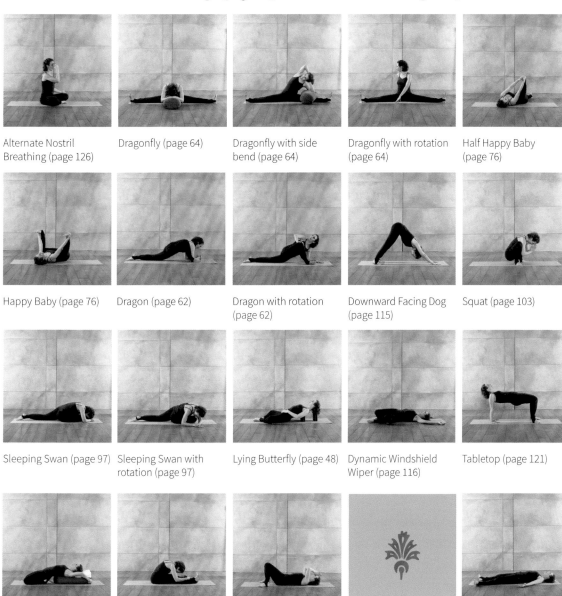

Alternate Nostril Breathing (page 126)

Dragonfly (page 64)

Dragonfly with side bend (page 64)

Dragonfly with rotation (page 64)

Half Happy Baby (page 76)

Happy Baby (page 76)

Dragon (page 62)

Dragon with rotation (page 62)

Downward Facing Dog (page 115)

Squat (page 103)

Sleeping Swan (page 97)

Sleeping Swan with rotation (page 97)

Lying Butterfly (page 48)

Dynamic Windshield Wiper (page 116)

Tabletop (page 121)

Saddle (page 90)

Caterpillar (page 51)

Resting Pose (page 89)

Cleansing Meditation (page 131)

Relaxed Supine Position (page 87)

❁ Foot Pain

Foot pain can be very limiting and is frequently associated with malpositioning or an uneven weight distribution on the feet. Frequent causes, for example, are shoes that are too narrow or small, poor shoe soles, or heels that are too high; additional causes include excess body weight, overloading, deformations that have developed in the foot, or weak foot muscles.

From a holistic perspective, the feet stand for stability and being rooted. It is important to always ground yourself and find your way back to your inner roots.

❁ **Possible questions for reflection are:**
Why do my roots need help?
Where am I not rooted?
What do I want to run away from?

From a TCM perspective, the therapy is directed towards the meridian where the main pain is located. Alternatively, the following entire functional circuits are treated:

- For complaints in the heel: bladder, pericardium, and kidney
- For complaints in the big toe joint: lungs, spleen, and liver
- For complaints in the ankle: triple warmer, kidney, and spleen
- For complaints in the side area of the foot: triple warmer, gallbladder, and bladder
- For complaints at the front of the foot: large intestine, stomach, and gallbladder
- For complaints in the Achilles tendon: kidney, bladder, and stomach

> ❁ This exercise stimulates the meridians in the feet, and makes the plantar fascia—the fascia in the sole of the foot—supple again. First, come into a comfortable standing position. Place a ball under the longitudinal arch of your right foot and move it left and right from the ankle. The heel should remain on the floor. Then place the ball and move the back part of the foot to and fro with the heel now lifted. Then place the ball under the toe joints, contract the toes on it, and spread them out again. Then lift and lower just the big toe, with the help of a finger if necessary. After that, keep the big toe on the ball and lift the other four toes. Finally, take the ball onto the inside of the foot and roll it up and down lengthways, going more towards the middle and finally to the outside. Then roll out the left foot. ❁

In addition to the **meridian massage** (page 36) and an extended foot massage, I recommend this **Yin Yoga sequence:**

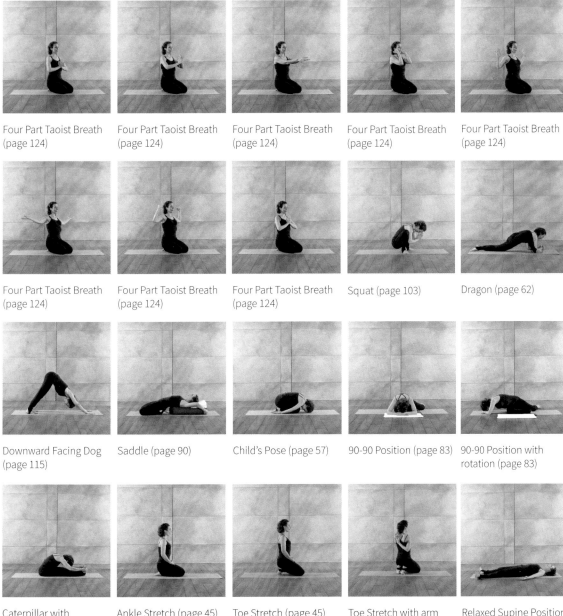

Four Part Taoist Breath (page 124)

Four Part Taoist Breath (page 124)

Four Part Taoist Breath (page 124)

Four Part Taoist Breath (page 124)

Four Part Taoist Breath (page 124)

Four Part Taoist Breath (page 124)

Four Part Taoist Breath (page 124)

Four Part Taoist Breath (page 124)

Squat (page 103)

Dragon (page 62)

Downward Facing Dog (page 115)

Saddle (page 90)

Child's Pose (page 57)

90-90 Position (page 83)

90-90 Position with rotation (page 83)

Caterpillar with acupressure point (page 52)

Ankle Stretch (page 45)

Toe Stretch (page 45)

Toe Stretch with arm and shoulder stretch (page 45)

Relaxed Supine Position (page 87)

❋ Headaches

Headaches are the second most common type of pain, after back pain. These are usually tension headaches, which result from pressure in the shoulder and neck area, or migraines. With acute tension headaches, Yin Yoga practice can often quickly bring relief, but for migraines it is much more about regular practice to promote the harmonious flow of the Chi.

From a holistic perspective, headaches often stand for brooding over emotional matters that have not been worked through or which have even been suppressed. This is fairly common in those cerebral people who have a lack of trust in their intuition.

❋ Possible questions for reflection are:

What emotions within me need to be lived more?
How can I have more trust in my intuition?
How can I better free myself from overthinking?

From the TCM perspective, a differentiation is made between fullness and emptiness headaches. With fullness, the pain tends to be sharp, explosive, pulsating, and clearly localized; for this, work on massaging the meridian against the flow of the meridian. For the empty type, it tends to be a duller and milder pain, in which case you massage in the flow of the meridian. The location of the pain decides which meridians are treated:

- For pain in the crown: liver, bladder, governing vessel, and gallbladder
- For pain in the temples: triple warmer and gallbladder
- For pain in the forehead: large intestine, stomach, governing vessel, and gallbladder
- For pain at the back of the head: bladder, small intestine, gallbladder, and governing vessel

❋ If you suffer frequently from headaches, magnesium can help as it has a relaxing and anti-convulsant effect. Very good sources of magnesium are amaranth, millet, bananas, green vegetables, oats, legumes, potatoes, nuts, kernels and seeds, cocoa, dried fruits, whole-grain products, and wild herbs. Headaches are also often due to a lack of fluids, so drinking is a top priority: I recommend two to three liters of (non-carbonated) water per day, and fresh mint tea is also good. Another proven remedy is turmeric, an old medicinal spice that supports the liver in detoxification and therefore counteracts detoxing symptoms. ❋

In addition to the **meridian massage** (page 36), I recommend this **Yin Yoga sequence:**

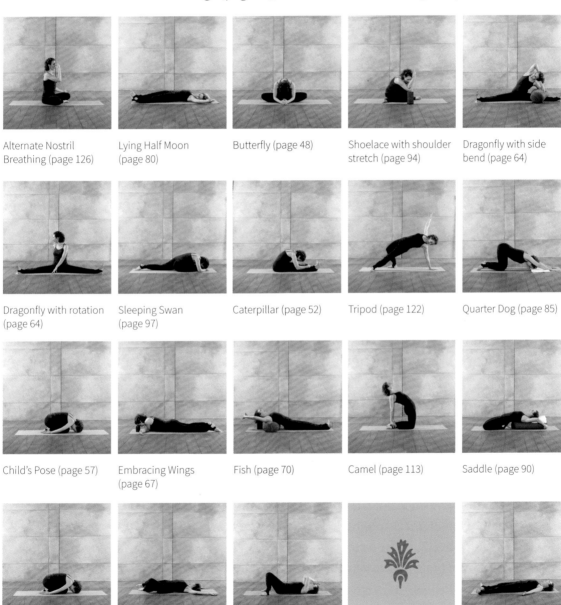

Alternate Nostril Breathing (page 126)

Lying Half Moon (page 80)

Butterfly (page 48)

Shoelace with shoulder stretch (page 94)

Dragonfly with side bend (page 64)

Dragonfly with rotation (page 64)

Sleeping Swan (page 97)

Caterpillar (page 52)

Tripod (page 122)

Quarter Dog (page 85)

Child's Pose (page 57)

Embracing Wings (page 67)

Fish (page 70)

Camel (page 113)

Saddle (page 90)

Child's Pose (page 57)

Twisted Twisted Roots (page 109)

Resting Pose (page 89)

Breath Meditation (page 131)

Relaxed Supine Position (page 87)

❀ Heavy Sweating

Sweating is a healthy process, and the body regulates its temperature in this way and excretes toxins. However, if you sweat excessively, you can often feel your quality of life is reduced, and you may be embarrassed by rings of sweat under the arms, beads of sweat on the forehead, or sweaty hands and feet.

From a holistic perspective, excessive sweating stands for a loss of vitality. As sweat comes through the skin to the exterior, it may mean that the person unconsciously tries to avoid close body contact. Ultimately, a form of anxiety sweating is possible, if you feel that you often have to be careful and cannot trust others. Yin Yoga practice can be very helpful for heavy sweating as it has a cooling effect on the body.

❀ **Possible questions for reflection are:**

What am I fearful of inside?

In what way do I over-exert myself, and what heated emotions am I suppressing?

From a TCM perspective, you can differentiate between two causes:

- If excess heat is coming from within, then it means recognizing the trigger and removing it.
- Sweating from exercise or sport regulates the body temperature and is therefore healthy and important.

For spontaneous sweating, treat the kidney (which carries the water out), spleen (which takes water from the food), lungs (which send water downwards and regulate the surface), and heart (which plays an important part in the emotional components of sweating).

❀ If you sweat a great deal, a large amount of non-carbonated water (best consumed at room temperature) should be drunk, to keep the fluid content of the body in balance. Sage tea is ideal, as it reduces sweating. As salt and electrolytes are also excreted via sweat, it is advisable to use natural original salt or rock salt, which contains more minerals and trace elements than table salt. Spices that are too hot can provoke sweating. On the other hand, food that is rich in zinc—such as yeast flakes, legumes, nuts, mushrooms, whole-grain bread (no wheat if you are gluten-sensitive), and vegetables—can slow down the formation of sweat. ❀

In addition to the **meridian massage** (page 36), which in this case treats the large intestine meridian against the direction of Chi flow, and the kidney (which treats the meridian in the direction of Chi flow), I recommend this **Yin Yoga sequence:**

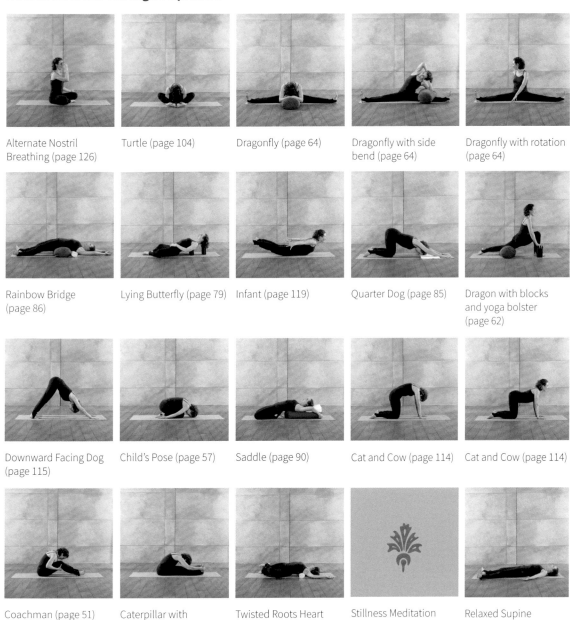

Alternate Nostril Breathing (page 126)

Turtle (page 104)

Dragonfly (page 64)

Dragonfly with side bend (page 64)

Dragonfly with rotation (page 64)

Rainbow Bridge (page 86)

Lying Butterfly (page 79)

Infant (page 119)

Quarter Dog (page 85)

Dragon with blocks and yoga bolster (page 62)

Downward Facing Dog (page 115)

Child's Pose (page 57)

Saddle (page 90)

Cat and Cow (page 114)

Cat and Cow (page 114)

Coachman (page 51)

Caterpillar with acupressure point page 51)

Twisted Roots Heart Opener (page 108)

Stillness Meditation (page 132)

Relaxed Supine Position (page 87)

❈ High Blood Pressure

High blood pressure is a common complaint in the West, which barely shows any symptoms initially and can therefore remain unrecognized and untreated for a long time. However, so-called hypertonia can have serious effects, including stroke or heart attack, and prevention is therefore essential. As high blood pressure can in many cases be attributed to an unhealthy lifestyle, those affected are urged to make a particular effort here.

From a holistic perspective, it is a slow process that ultimately causes high blood pressure. Many factors combine that lead to the condition.

❈ **Possible questions for reflection are:**
What is causing me too much pressure in my life?
Where do I put too much pressure on myself?
What is close to my heart and how can I live it more?

❈ With high blood pressure, it is important to reduce excess body weight, to give up stimulants such as tobacco, nicotine, and alcohol, to exercise, and to reduce negative stress. Diet also plays an important part. Polyunsaturated fatty acids—such as in walnut and linseed oil, as well as oily fish, for example—can work against high triglyceride and cholesterol values, and can prevent arteriosclerosis (sediments in the vessels). Olive oil and avocados contain valuable oleic acid, a monounsaturated fatty acid, which can help lower harmful LDL cholesterol levels and can increase protective HDL cholesterol. Legumes and whole-grain products provide fiber, and can also have a cholesterol-lowering and vascular-protecting effect. Salt can also increase blood pressure in many patients. If you are sensitive to salt, salty foods should be avoided; try seasoning with fresh herbs instead. Generally a vegetarian diet is recommended for most, as fruit and vegetables are low in sodium but score high with many minerals that regulate the water-electrolyte balance of the body. Fatty dairy products, industrially produced foods, meat, and sausage products should only be consumed occasionally, for they contain several ingredients that can lead to arteriosclerosis—including sodium, saturated fatty acids, trans fats, and cholesterol. ❈

Interestingly, **TCM** does not know the illness of high blood pressure. Here, it is much more a Chi blockage in the liver that is assumed. Therapies therefore focus on the liver, the large intestine, and the pericardium. In the case of excess body weight, the stomach is also treated, and for long-lasting stress, the kidney.

In addition to the **meridian massage** (page 36), I recommend this **Yin Yoga sequence:**

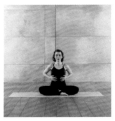

Full Breathing with extended exhalation (page 128)

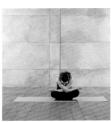

Easy Pose with arm and shoulder stretch (page 66)

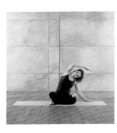

Square with side bend (page 101)

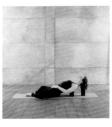

Lying Butterfly (page 79)

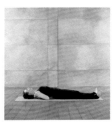

Twisted Arms (page 105)

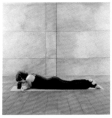

Embracing Wings (page 67)

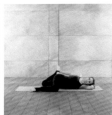

Cat Pulling Its Tail (page 50)

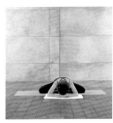

Dragonfly (page 64)

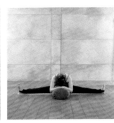

Frog* (page 71)

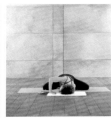

Frog with rotation* (page 71)

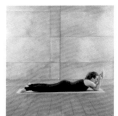

Sphinx with shoulder stretch (page 99)

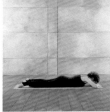

Resting Forward Pose (page 88)

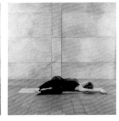

Twisted Roots (page 106)

Stillness Meditation (page 132)

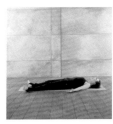

Relaxed Supine Position (page 87)

* In case of high blood pressure, when in Frog, please rest your head slightly raised, perhaps on a block.

✿ Hollow Back

Hollow back has to do with poor posture, with a strongly pronounced lordosis (curvature of the spine in the direction of the abdominal wall) of the lumbar spine. Hollow back does not have to lead to complaints, as the thoracic spine frequently compensates for this posture and comes into a stronger kyphosis (curvature rearward, towards the back). However, if the lordosis causes pain, Yin Yoga practice can counteract this beautifully by focusing more on forward bends. With Yang Yoga, on the other hand, the strengthening of the back is important. In Yin Yoga, you always go consciously into a passive hollow back position and into a passive rounding of the spine—to address the long fascia chains, on the one hand, and to promote the natural flexibility of the spine on the other. As the Yin Yoga exercises can always be assisted by using props and can be adapted individually, you should be able to go into these positions safely.

From a holistic perspective, malposition of the spine stands for bending too much or distortion. Those affected frequently try to please everyone and they lack inner alignment.

✿ **Possible questions for reflection are:**
For whom or what am I distorting myself?
What is my own truth?
How can I live out my own needs more?

In TCM, the treatment for hollow back involves the kidney, liver, gallbladder, and possibly the spleen for muscle and tendon strength.

> ✿ For complaints caused by hollow back, a fascia exercise with two small balls may help. Place the balls in a net or sock; lie on your back and place the balls next to one another under your lumbar spine so that they are to the right and left of it. Prop yourself up with your lower arms on the floor, place the feet on the floor, and move slowly to and fro on the balls. If the balls are soft, you can then position the ball-roller lengthways on the spine and roll from left to right (I would not recommend this with very hard fascia balls, though). Also, you can use the balls individually, or place them further apart if you wish. Alternatively, you can do this exercise against the wall while standing. ✿

In addition to the **meridian massage** (page 36), I recommend this **Yin Yoga sequence:**

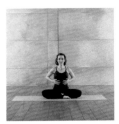

Full Breathing
(Tip: when lying with feet on floor) (page 128)

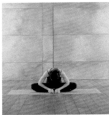

Butterfly with acupressure point (page 48)

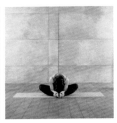

Turtle with acupressure point (page 104)

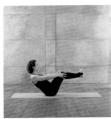

Boat (page 112)

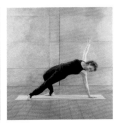

Tripod (page 122)

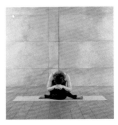

Shoelace (page 94)

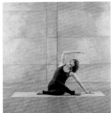

Shoelace with side bend (page 94)

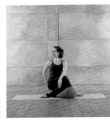

Shoelace with rotation (page 94)

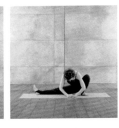

Crane (page 58)

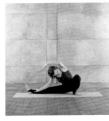

Crane with side bend (page 58)

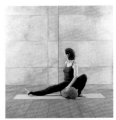

Crane with rotation (page 58)

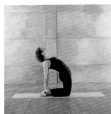

Camel (page 113)

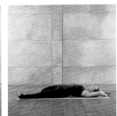

Half Saddle (page 90)

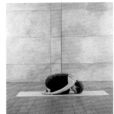

Child's Pose (page 57)

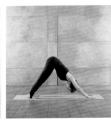

Downward Facing Dog (page 115)

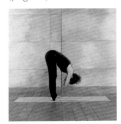

Standing Forward Bend (page 60)

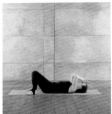

Resting Pose (page 89)

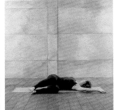

Twisted Roots (page 106)

Stillness Meditation (page 132)

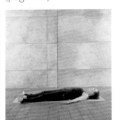

Relaxed Supine Position (page 87)

❀ Hunched Back

Hunchback is a misalignment whereby the shoulder blades push forward and upward and kyphosis (curvature of the spine outwards) of the thoracic spine is very apparent. If the hunched back causes pain in the neck and headaches are triggered as a result, this can be counteracted very nicely through Yin Yoga practice by focusing on backbends. In Yang Yoga, strengthening the abdomen and the whole front of the body is also important. In Yin Yoga, you keep going consciously into a passive hollow back, as well as into a passive rounding of the spine, in order to address the long fascial chains on the one hand, and to promote the natural flexibility of the spine on the other. As the Yin Yoga exercises can always be assisted by using props and can be adapted individually, you should be able to carry out these positions safely and without any concerns.

From a holistic perspective, a hunched back stands for problems that weigh you down. Some people defer to avoid confrontations. Inner peace is often lacking and you may feel torn.

❀ **Possible questions for reflection are:**
Where in my life am I lacking support, and how can I acquire it?
Can I meet confrontations with self-confidence?
How can I make peace with my past problems?

In TCM, hunchback is treated via the bladder and small intestine meridian.

❀ A fascia exercise using two balls can alleviate complaints caused by a hunched back. Place the balls in a net or sock; lie on your back and place the balls under your thoracic spine so that they are to the right and left of it. Support your head in your folded hands, then place your feet on the floor, lift your pelvis, and move slowly to and fro on the balls. If the balls are soft, you can then place the ball-roller lengthways next to the spine and roll from right to left or circle the shoulder blades (I would not recommend this with very hard fascia balls, though). Decide by feeling into it whether to also use the balls individually, or whether to place them a little further apart or lower. Alternatively, you can do the exercise standing against a wall. ❀

In addition to the **meridian massage** (page 36), I recommend this **Yin Yoga sequence:**

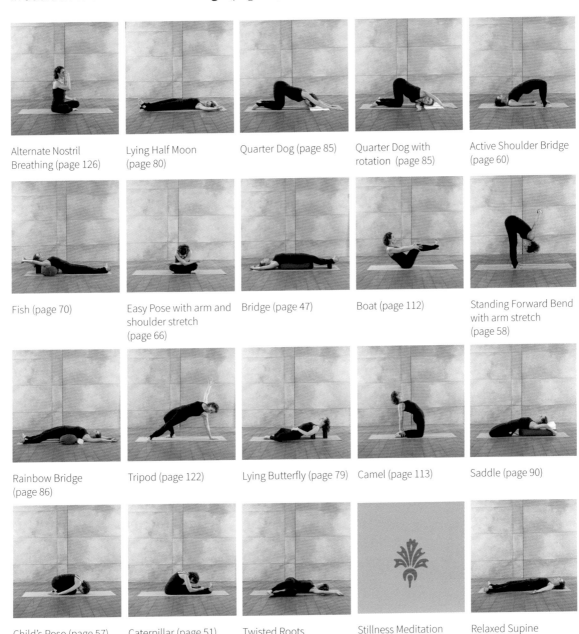

Alternate Nostril
Breathing (page 126)

Lying Half Moon
(page 80)

Quarter Dog (page 85)

Quarter Dog with
rotation (page 85)

Active Shoulder Bridge
(page 60)

Fish (page 70)

Easy Pose with arm and
shoulder stretch
(page 66)

Bridge (page 47)

Boat (page 112)

Standing Forward Bend
with arm stretch
(page 58)

Rainbow Bridge
(page 86)

Tripod (page 122)

Lying Butterfly (page 79)

Camel (page 113)

Saddle (page 90)

Child's Pose (page 57)

Caterpillar (page 51)

Twisted Roots
(page 106)

Stillness Meditation
(page 132)

Relaxed Supine
Position (page 87)

❧ Infertility

The unfulfilled wish for a child affects many more couples today than it did in the past. Possible causes may be environmental pollution, less nutrition in our food, a lack of care for the self, or negative stress. What should not be underestimated is the high level of expectation for a healthy woman to be able to become pregnant quickly and with no problems.

From a holistic perspective, pregnancy occurs when the parents are ready to accept a new soul, and when the soul decides upon these parents.

❧ Possible questions for reflection are:

Am I really ready for a child in the depth of my being?
Do I look after myself well enough? Do I have enough strength and energy to look after another person?
How can I better let go and trust?

TCM treats the kidney, heart, and uterus in the event of the unfulfilled wish for a child, as well as the connections to the eight extraordinary vessels (see page 26) and the liver, stomach, and spleen.

❧ In TCM as well as in Ayurveda, couples who want a child are advised to detoxify so that the unborn baby has the best preconditions for being healthy. This recommendation also applies in the case of the unfulfilled wish for a child. Detoxification includes a vitamin and nutrient-rich diet with a lot of fresh fruit, vegetables, salad, nuts, seeds, wholegrain products, herbs and wild herbs, potatoes, spices, coconut oil, sesame oil or olive oil, non-carbonated water, and herbal tea. These also usually counteract excess body weight by themselves—another important factor that may play a part in infertility. Stimulants such as caffeine, nicotine, alcohol, and sugar disrupt the detoxification process, and should be reduced as far as possible at this time. Intestinal cleansing treatments are also recommended. As stress may also be responsible for infertility, Yin Yoga practice is ideal as it can have a positive effect on the entire vegetative nervous system. ❧

In addition to the **meridian massage** (page 36), I recommend this **Yin Yoga sequence:**

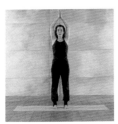

Energy Breathing
(page 127)

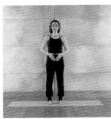

Energy Breathing
(page 127)

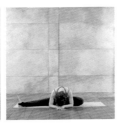

Half Dragonfly (page 64)

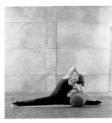

Dragonfly with side
bend (page 64)

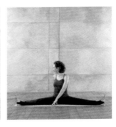

Dragonfly with rotation
(page 64)

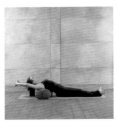

Fish (page 70)

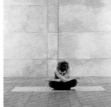

Easy Pose with arm
and shoulder stretch
(page 66)

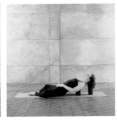

Lying Butterfly (page 79)

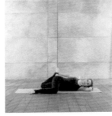

Cat Pulling Its Tail
(page 50)

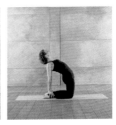

Camel (page 113)

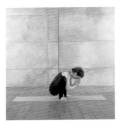

Squat (page 103)

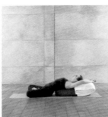

Half Lying Lotus
(page 75)

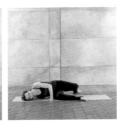

Open Wings (page 84)

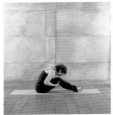

Coachman (page 51)

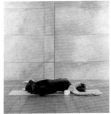

Twisted Roots Heart
Opener (page 108)

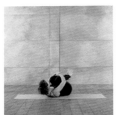

Folded Pose (page 117)

Stomach Massage with
hands or ball (page 43)

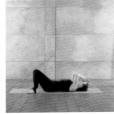

Resting Pose (page 89)

Protective Meditation
(page 132)

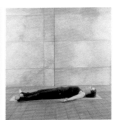

Relaxed Supine Position
(page 87)

❇ Knee Pain

Knees can be very prone to pain, particularly in athletes or older people whose joints are suffering from wear and tear. Knee pain is also often associated with the iliotibial band, the fascia on the outside of the leg, which can be too tense. It is naturally very firm to stabilize the hip joints. Therefore, the following sequence is not only directed to the relevant meridians but also stretches the iliotibial band in many positions. Yin Yoga generally can have a very positive effect on the joints. If the suggested sequence is too difficult—depending on the degree of severity of the pain—then as an alternative you should try the sequence for limited movement (see page 181), which includes a chair and therefore exerts less pressure on the knees. Of couse, you can also simply keep the exercises shorter, or use more props at any time in order to avoid any uncomfortable pressure or pain in the knee area.

From a holistic perspective, the knees have something to do with humility: we go onto our knees when we surrender. However, we also need the knees to be able to run upright, and likewise they therefore also stand for our life path.

❇ Possible questions for reflection are:
What circumstances in my life put pressure on my knees?
Am I meeting the challenges on my life path boldly and with drive?
Am I following my life path and listening to my inner voice?

In TCM, the meridians of kidney, liver, stomach, spleen, and gallbladder are treated when there is knee pain.

❇ Again, a rolling-out exercise for the fascia can be helpful for knee pain. You will need two balls placed in a net or sock. Come onto all fours and place the ball-roller crosswise under your right knee. Just hold the pressure to start with, and then begin to move your knee forwards and backwards. Then take one ball out of the roll, lie on the mat, angle the right leg, and place the ball in the back of your right knee. Raise the lower leg close to the upper leg, thereby massaging the back of the knee. Roll the right knee out for a few minutes and then change sides. ❇

In addition to the **meridian massage** (page 36), I recommend this **Yin Yoga sequence:**

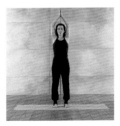

Energy Breathing
(page 127)

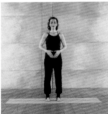

Energy Breathing
(page 127)

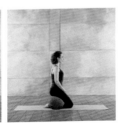

Ankle Stretch with Yoga
bolster (page 45)

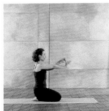

Ankle Stretch with finger
stretch (page 45)

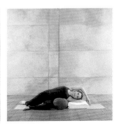

Lying Banana
(page 78)

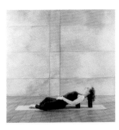

Lying Butterfly (page 79)

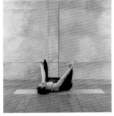

Happy Baby (page 76)

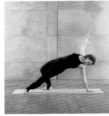

Tripod (page 122)

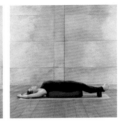

Bridge (page 47)

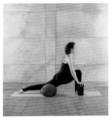

Dragon with blocks
and yoga bolster
(page 62)

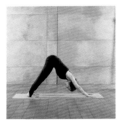

Downward Facing Dog
(page 115)

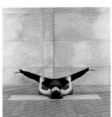

Dragonfly in back
position (page 64)

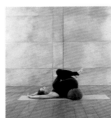

Eye of the Needle
(page 68)

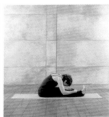

Eye of the Needle with
rotation (page 68)

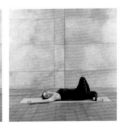

Caterpillar (page 51)

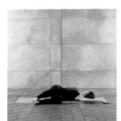

Twisted Roots
(page 106)

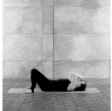

Resting Pose (page 89)

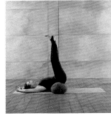

Seagrass (page 92)

Stillness Meditation
(page 132)

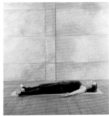

Relaxed Supine Position
(page 87)

❧ Limited Movement in Old Age

It is important to keep moving and do physical activity in old age. For example, if health limitations lead to poor and restrictive posture, the body adjusts accordingly: the muscles degenerate, and the metabolism of the bones and joints is reduced, too. Those who remain active can keep the body supple and counteract the changes that come with age. However, there is no place here for a performance mentality. Many people believe that all exercises have to be carried out perfectly, and if that does not work out, then they often drop out completely. Please do not think like this. In Yin Yoga, in particular, it is not all about perfection but much more about stimulating through stretching and encouraging the flow of energy. If an exercise seems very difficult, then adjust it until it can be carried out more easily. The exercise images shown here should be viewed with this in mind: they demonstrate various options, but no leg has to be extended in exactly that way, and any supporting cushion is welcome. The limits of your own body are the benchmark, and therefore positions may be adapted to what is possible for you.

From a holistic perspective, the aging process does not mean regretting lost youth or giving in to aches and pains. It is important to adapt the practice of your exercises to your current requirements. A chair can serve well if exercising on the floor seems too difficult. With Yin Yoga, it is all about feeling the stretch and the relaxing effect, and not about impressing anybody in a position.

❧ Possible questions for reflection are:
Am I able to accept my age well?
What can I do to get the best out of this stage of life?
Where have I become rigid or immobile in my mind?

❧ Older people usually do not have such a good appetite anymore, which is a very natural impulse as the metabolism slows down. For this reason, care should be taken to select high-quality, nutritious foods, as smaller amounts are required. Another important point is that it is essential to continue to drink sufficiently, even if you do not feel thirsty. Here is a small trick to avoid dehydration: preparing two large bottles of non-carbonated water or a large pot of tea in the morning will be an automatic reminder to drink regularly throughout the day. ❧

From a TCM perspective, the prenatal kidney energy (in Chinese, "Jing") decreases, as does the postnatal energy of the spleen and stomach. The consequences of everyday life also become noticeable with a variety of stress factors. From the age of fifty, an additional lung Chi weakness often occurs, particularly with smokers and passive smokers. The worsening of the memory can also be attributed to a weakness of the kidney energy, as can the increasing wear and tear on the bony musculoskeletal system. The best treatment for elderly people is therefore the kidney, spleen, stomach, lungs, and liver in particular. To strengthen the Chi of the kidneys, our treasure trove, you can place a hot water bottle on the lower stomach and lower back every evening.

In addition to the **meridian massage** (page 36), I recommend this **Yin Yoga sequence:**

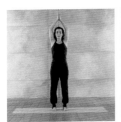
Energy Breathing (page 127)

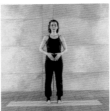
Energy Breathing (page 127)

Breath Meditation (page 131)

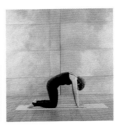
Cat and Cow (page 114)

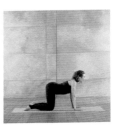
Cat and Cow (page 114)

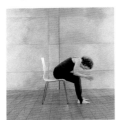
Gentle Dangling Pose with chair (page 53)

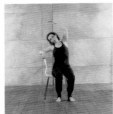
Side Bend with chair (page 53)

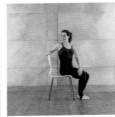
Rotation with chair (page 53)

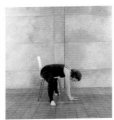
Hip Opener (Inner) with chair (page 53)

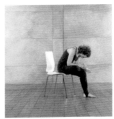
Hip Opener (Outer) with chair (page 54)

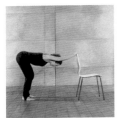
Backbend with chair (page 53)

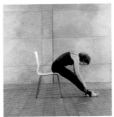
Long Dangling Pose with chair (page 53)

Meridian Tapping Massage (page 41)

Stillness meditation (page 132)

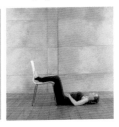
Relaxed Supine Position with chair (page 54)

❈ Menopause

During menopause, a woman's hormones adjust and her body changes gradually. Most women notice these changes between the ages of forty and fifty-five. They are often accompanied by unpleasant symptoms such as hot flushes, irritability, aggression, lethargy, feeling faint, gaining weight, or hair loss. The inner attitude of the woman also has a major effect on how the menopause progresses. If she is positive about this phase of life, the typical menopause complaints are much less severe or may not even be perceived as such. You can see this in cultures that celebrate this transition instead of meeting it critically.

Many women question themselves and their own lives intensively during this period, and may also concentrate more on themselves again, as they have reached a very stable phase of life and no

❈ Vegetarians and vegans usually have fewer menopausal complaints than omnivores. If you suffer badly from hot flushes, etc., then you should avoid animal products as far as possible for a while. Some women are also helped by phytoestrogens, secondary plant substances with a hormonal effect. The best-known representative of this is isoflavone, which is found in red clover and soy in particular. Asians seem to benefit from this more (and Europeans a little less, probably because they have a different intestinal flora and metabolize soy differently). The lignans contained especially in flax seed, legumes, vegetables, whole grains, and fruit (particularly in pomegranates) may also have a balancing effect. I would not recommend taking highly concentrated phytoestrogens supplements, however, as they can have unwanted side effects. On the other hand, women going through menopause should pay particular attention to their bone health and make sure they intake a sufficient supply of calcium and vitamin D, as a lack of estrogen can also lead to osteoporosis. Good supplies of calcium include seaweed, dandelion, cabbage, fennel, nuts, almonds, poppy seeds, and sesame seeds. Unfortunately, the vitamin D requirement is not just covered by nutrition, as it is mainly formed in the skin via UV-B radiation. Moderate sunbathing is fantastic to increase vitamin D levels. However, if there is a proven lack in vitamin D sufficiency (there is a blood test for this), a supplement is recommended. During the fall and winter months, I take a supplement myself because the sun is not high enough in the European countries to give us sufficient vitamin D. ❈

longer have to—or want to—subject themselves to the pressures of society as they might have in the past. Mothers, in particular, will have done an amazing and brilliant job for many years (and given a considerable amount of themselves, through pregnancy and the raising of children), and they should really enjoy having more time to themselves once their children are independent. In this phase, plans and wishes that women have kept on the back burner for some time should now be implemented and enjoyed before possible physical limitations might start to become apparent and these opportunities would no longer be possible.

As the Yin energy should be nurtured during menopause, Yin Yoga is naturally ideal here. It also has a cooling effect, which can have a very favorable influence on hot flushes. Many women intuitively gravitate to calmer styles of yoga in these years, as they no longer have the strength or willingness for active types of yoga. However, many use it consciously as a form of balance to neutralize the excessive Yang, which has often built up in the first half of life.

From a holistic perspective, menopause is a time when a woman questions herself again. She is starting the second half of her life and losing her fertility at a physical level, which can also give her new freedom. Although it is frequently devalued in the West, the midlife crisis, which men may also experience, should not be viewed negatively. This upheaval should really be a welcome opportunity to set new objectives or venture into a change of direction—to be able to look back on a fulfilled life and to have no regrets about not having lived life to the fullest.

❋ **Possible questions for reflection are:**
Have I sufficiently accepted my femininity?
How can I live out my intellectual and spiritual sides more?
Am I ready to move on to new topics and tasks?

In TCM, there are two conflicting notions. One assumes that with menopause there is a lack of Yin, which allows the Yang to increase excessively, and the other presumes that the Chi dynamic is out of control. In modern China, the "School of Yin nourishment" dominates, so that it is treated as follows:
- For hot flushes worsened by stress: kidney, liver, and large intestine; if sleep disturbances also occur, the heart and liver as well
- For hot flushes with heavy sweats: kidney
- For restlessness, sleep disturbances, and palpitations: heart, liver, and kidney; if there is also faintness, then liver, spleen, and stomach as well

In addition to the **meridian massage** (page 36), I recommend this **Yin Yoga sequence:**

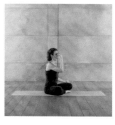

Alternate Nostril Breathing (page 126)

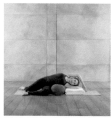

Lying Banana (page 78)

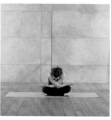

Lying Butterfly (page 79)

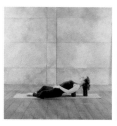

Easy Pose with arm and shoulder stretch (page 66)

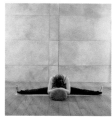

Dragonfly (page 64)

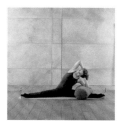

Dragonfly with side bend (page 64)

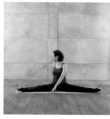

Dragonfly with rotation (page 64)

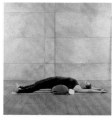

Rainbow Bridge (page 86)

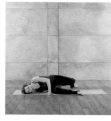

Open Wings (page 84)

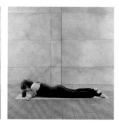

Embracing Wings (page 67)

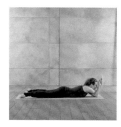

Sphinx with shoulder stretch (page 99)

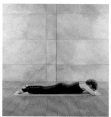

Resting Forward Pose (page 88)

Stomach Massage with ball (page 43)

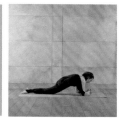

Dragon (page 62)

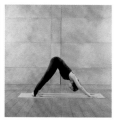

Downward Facing Dog (page 115)

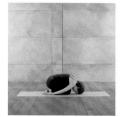

Child's Pose with bolster (page 57)

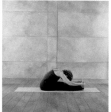

Caterpillar with acupressure point (page 51)

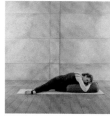

Sitting Twisted Roots (page 96)

Stillness Meditation (page 132)

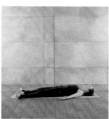

Relaxed Supine Position (page 87)

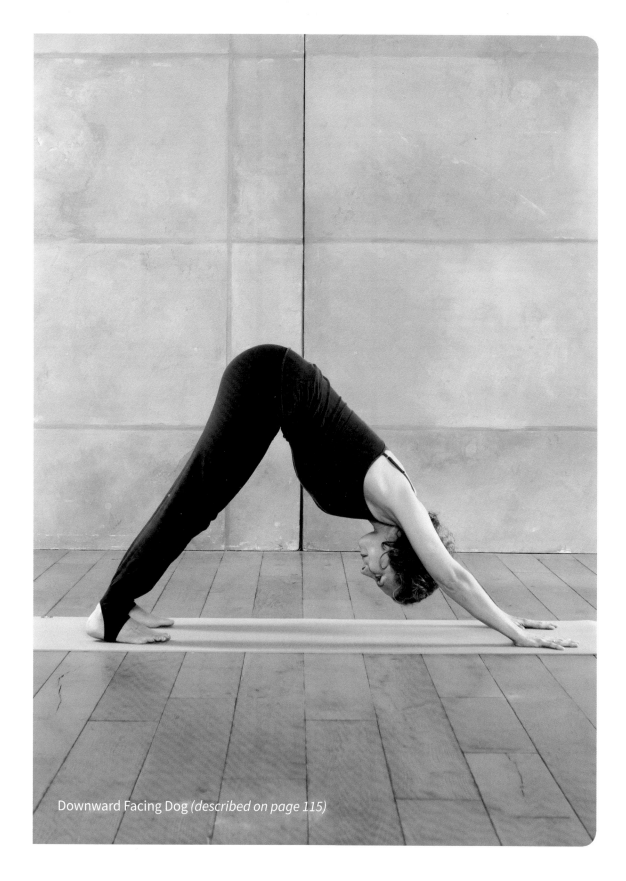

Downward Facing Dog *(described on page 115)*

❧ Menstruation Problems and PMS

Menstruation problems arise either before or during menstruation and can be very stressful. The most frequent have to do with menstrual pain or pre-menstrual syndrome (PMS). Menstrual pain occurs due to muscle contractions in the uterus, which has to contract to be able to shed the lining of the womb. PMS symptoms are numerous; they range from water collecting in the body and tightness of the breasts to changes in the skin, cramps in the lower abdomen, and digestion complaints, to tiredness or irritability. PMS emerges up to two weeks before menstruation and ends with the onset of bleeding. Many women also feel their personal freedom is limited during this time, as they want to be close to a bathroom if there is heavy bleeding, in order to be able to change their tampons or pads. Menstrual cups are a great option. They are produced using medical silicone and are available in various sizes and degrees of hardness, so that women can select a suitable model for their individual needs. The cups catch a great deal more blood than other monthly hygiene products and

❧ For menstruation complaints and PMS, those affected may wish to try magnesium-rich foods, as is the case with headaches; in this respect the same recommendations apply here: amaranth, millet, bananas, green vegetables, oats, legumes, potatoes, nuts, kernels, seeds, cocoa, whole-grain products, dried fruits, and wild herbs ensure a good supply of magnesium. While magnesium relaxes and eases cramps, additional calcium can also alleviate complaints—calcium regulates the irritability of muscle and nerve cells. There is a great deal of calcium, for example, in seaweed, stinging nettles, broccoli, fennel, green cabbage, savoy cabbage, dandelion, nuts and kernels (particularly almonds), seeds (particularly poppy and sesame), eggs, and dairy products. It's important to know that various substances, such as phosphate (for example, in soft cheese, cola drinks, and sausage products), oxalic acid (for example, in spinach, beetroot, rhubarb, and chocolate), or dietary fibers can restrict the uptake of calcium or even absorb it, and should therefore not be eaten in conjunction with calcium-rich foods. Besides this, salt or too much coffee encourages the excretion of calcium. Studies also indicate that dairy products are not an optimal source of calcium: indeed, they contain relatively large amounts of the important minerals but, due to the phosphate and protein content of the milk, they cannot be utilized optimally. ❧

are very durable, which saves a lot of trash. Many women with heavy bleeding can even experience peaceful and dry nights where they no longer need to get up and change their protection, thanks to menstrual cups.

From a holistic perspective, menstruation complaints are associated with a decreasing acceptance of one's own femininity, and possibly also with anger and feelings of guilt. The period of menstruation is seen as a cleaning ritual, and in the first few days a woman may indulge in more rest and recovery. For mothers, it should be natural to pass on to their daughters that menstruation is a natural process which should not evoke negative feelings. Young girls therefore learn to deal more naturally with their femininity; this mainly has a positive effect on their further development and the subsequent years of fertility. Women with a negative attitude to menstruation suffer more significantly and frequently from menstrual problems and also suffer worse symptoms in menopause. In some countries, women are given "permission" to consciously withdraw during menstruation to support their body in the purification, and so they may indulge in a break. Such rituals change the perspective on the process and steer it in a positive direction—instead of framing it as a source of embarrassment, as is often still the case in the West.

❋ **Possible questions for reflection are:**
Can I completely accept my essence as a woman and the feminine energies?
Am I happy on the path I have chosen?
Do I implement my own creativity, or do I simply bend to others?
How can I trust in the flow of life better?

TCM differentiates between two different conditions here and treats them accordingly:
- For pain shortly before and at the start of menstruation: liver, spleen, and stomach
- For pain at the end of menstruation: conception vessel, spleen, stomach, and liver
- For tenderness in the breasts: triple warmer, stomach, liver, gallbladder, and—for emotional stress causing feelings of pressure in the chest—the pericardium as well
- For mood swings, feelings of frustration, depressive moods, and irritability: liver, large intestine, bladder, and pericardium

In addition to the **meridian massage** (page 36), I recommend this **Yin Yoga sequence:**

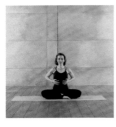

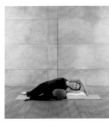

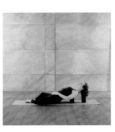

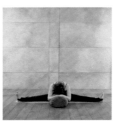

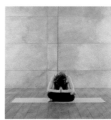

Full Breathing
(Tip: lie with hands
on the stomach)
(page 128)

Lying Banana (page 78)

Lying Butterfly (page 79)

Dragonfly (page 64)

Square (page 101)

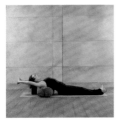

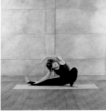

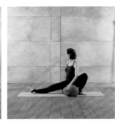

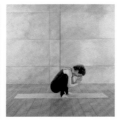

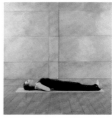

Fish (page 70)

Crane with side bend
(page 58)

Crane with rotation
(page 58)

Squat (page 103)

Twisted Arms
(page 105)

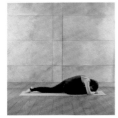

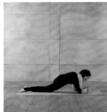

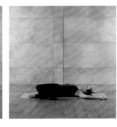

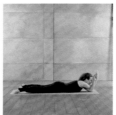

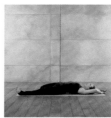

Sleeping Swan
(page 97)

Dragon (page 62)

Dynamic Windshield
Wiper (page 116)

Sphinx with shoulder
stretch (page 99)

Half Saddle (page 90)

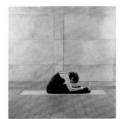

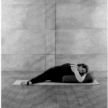

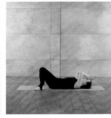

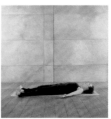

Caterpillar (page 51)

Sitting Twisted Roots
(page 96)

Resting Pose (page 89)

Breath Meditation
(page 131)

Relaxed Supine Position
(page 87)

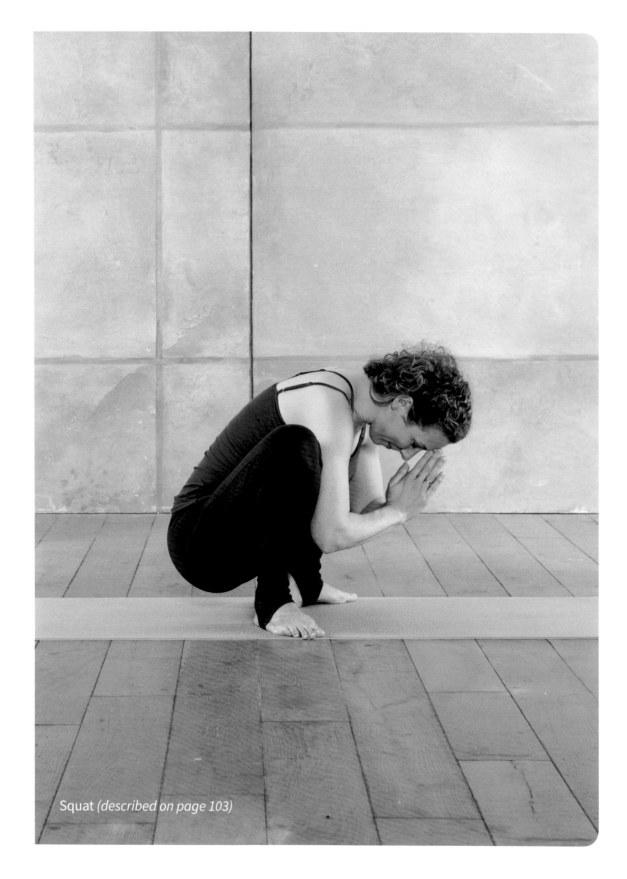

Squat *(described on page 103)*

❧ Neck Pain

The shoulder and neck area is a weak spot of the spine, and many Westerners complain of tension in the neck and back. One of the main causes of this is hours of sitting in a bent position on chairs. If someone does this each day, the body gradually adapts and then it is high time to take consistent counter measures. Bending forward in Yin Yoga can be very good to stretch the neck area. If the neck is very tense it may feel fairly unpleasant at the beginning. However, this should not discourage you from continuing to practice it. Work consciously with more calm and attention, use more props to rest your head accordingly, or activate your neck muscles any time by turning your head left and right or up and down a few times.

From a holistic perspective, the neck stands for self-confidence. As it can be assumed that energy flows through the spine, the energy flow is often blocked here when there is chronic neck tension. The throat chakra is located in this area (see page 27), and this is our center of communication. It Is also important to come to terms with your own past and work through any setbacks you have experienced.

❋ **Possible questions for reflection are:**
Who or what is weighing me down?
What do I still need to communicate?
Am I self-confident, or do I bend for others?

In TCM it is the gallbladder, bladder, small intestine, and triple warmer that are treated in the event of neck problems.

> ❧ If you have painful tension in the neck area, the following fascia exercise can help. You need two small balls for this, which you can place in a sock or net; position them slightly raised on a yoga block or a book. Then lie on your back and place the ball-roller crossways under your neck. Move your head slowly up and down, to and fro, and make small circles, as though forming small figure eights with your head while lying down. Roll out your neck for as long as it feels good. Do this daily if you like. ❧

In addition to the **meridian massage** (page 36), I recommend this **Yin Yoga sequence.** Please assume a comfortable sitting position before starting and after completing the sequence, and feel into your neck consciously for a few moments.

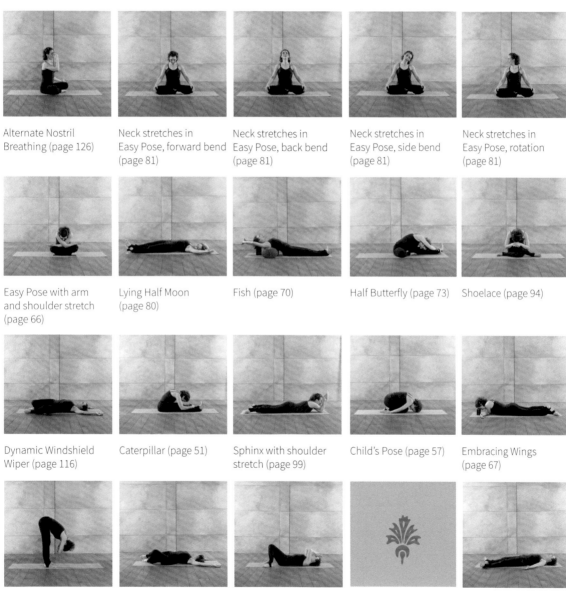

Alternate Nostril Breathing (page 126)

Neck stretches in Easy Pose, forward bend (page 81)

Neck stretches in Easy Pose, back bend (page 81)

Neck stretches in Easy Pose, side bend (page 81)

Neck stretches in Easy Pose, rotation (page 81)

Easy Pose with arm and shoulder stretch (page 66)

Lying Half Moon (page 80)

Fish (page 70)

Half Butterfly (page 73)

Shoelace (page 94)

Dynamic Windshield Wiper (page 116)

Caterpillar (page 51)

Sphinx with shoulder stretch (page 99)

Child's Pose (page 57)

Embracing Wings (page 67)

Standing Forward Bend (page 60)

Twisted Twisted Roots (page 109)

Resting Pose (page 89)

Breath Meditation (page 131)

Relaxed Supine Position (page 87)

❊ Respiratory Problems

Respiratory problems often present in the form of breathing difficulties or shortness of breath. An adult normally breathes on average twelve to eighteen times per minute. Yoga practitioners often manage with six to eight breaths as they practice certain techniques that train deep breathing. Environmental influences, psychological problems, and illnesses such as asthma can also restrict the breathing.

From a holistic perspective, there is a difference between problems with inhalation and exhalation: difficulties with inhalation are linked in the figurative sense with topics such as rejection and non-acceptance, and problems exhaling relate to difficulties in giving up and letting go.

❊ Possible questions for reflection are:

What is stopping me from breathing?
What am I unable to accept?
What am I unable to let go of?

In TCM it is usually the lungs, spleen, and kidneys that are treated.

❊ Respiratory problems can be influenced positively not only through yoga or sports, but also with the right choice of nutrition. A diet that is low in salt can improve lung function and alleviate possible narrowing of the bronchial tubes. The same recommendations apply as for allergies (see page 138), as allergic reactions frequently occur in the area of the respiratory tract. Histamine plays an important role here. If the body comes into contact with an allergen, more of this messenger substance is released, provoking the immune reaction. A high intake of vitamin C—for example, dark green vegetables, peppers, or parsley—can help reduce the distribution of histamine. Sauerkraut or citrus fruits are less suitable here; they are rich in vitamin C but are a source of histamine in themselves, and tend also to stimulate the release of histamine. Additionally, it is advisable to cut out dairy products, as they often have a congesting effect and can therefore hamper the breathing. ❊

In addition to the **meridian massage** (page 36), I recommend this **Yin Yoga sequence:**

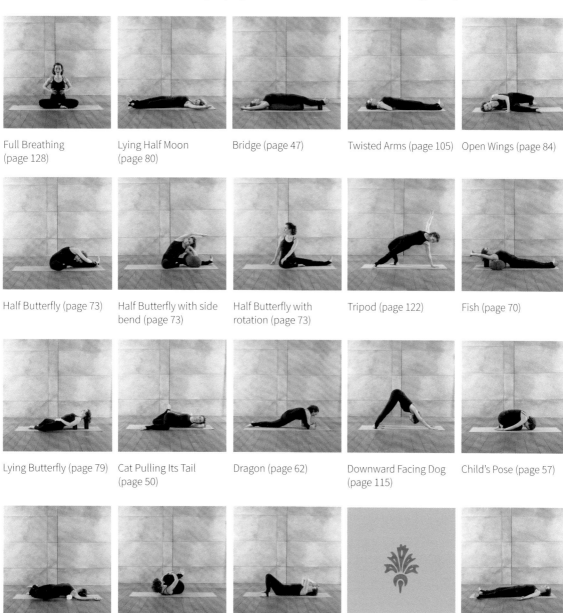

Full Breathing
(page 128)

Lying Half Moon
(page 80)

Bridge (page 47)

Twisted Arms (page 105)

Open Wings (page 84)

Half Butterfly (page 73)

Half Butterfly with side
bend (page 73)

Half Butterfly with
rotation (page 73)

Tripod (page 122)

Fish (page 70)

Lying Butterfly (page 79)

Cat Pulling Its Tail
(page 50)

Dragon (page 62)

Downward Facing Dog
(page 115)

Child's Pose (page 57)

Twisted Roots Heart
Opener (page 108)

Folded Pose (page 117)

Resting Pose (page 89)

Breath Meditation
(page 131)

Relaxed Supine Position
(page 87)

❧ Shoulder Pain

The shoulder joint is the most mobile of all the joints; it does not have a deep socket and primarily holds the humeral head in position via ligaments, tendons, and muscles. The shoulder is therefore very susceptible to injury, and shoulder pain, like neck pain, is very widespread. Calcifications and inflammations often occur, but arthrosis and poor posture can also cause shoulder pain. In many Yin Yoga exercises, the shoulders are included so that the painful areas can get energized and be regenerated. Please place blocks or other props under your hands or arms if the stretches feel too intense.

From a holistic perspective, shoulder pain stands for too much of a burden or too much responsibility on the shoulders. Emotional hurt can also be a reason—we intuitively pull the shoulders up and forward to protect the heart area.

❋ **Possible questions for reflection are:**
Who or what is weighing on my shoulders?
How can I pass on more responsibility or tasks to others?
How can I indulge more in rest or time out?

In TCM, for shoulder pain the large intestine, small intestine, triple warmer, gallbladder, and stomach are treated. A remote point that is also suitable for shoulder pain is the Stomach 38 acupressure point. It is located in the middle of the lower leg, between the lower edge of the knee cap and the outer ankle, a thumb's width outside the shin.

> ❋ As shoulder pain is often related to the fascia, a fascia exercise with two balls can be a good option to alleviate this. Lie on your back and place the balls under your shoulder blades. Place your head on your folded hands, put your feet on the floor, raise your pelvis, and move very slowly to and fro on the balls, or start circular movements. Position the balls above the shoulder blades, then on the inside next to the spine, and finally on the outside and underneath the shoulder blades. Roll out as long as it feels good. Alternatively, you can also do this exercise standing in front of a wall. ❋

In addition to the **meridian massage** (page 36), I recommend this **Yin Yoga sequence:**

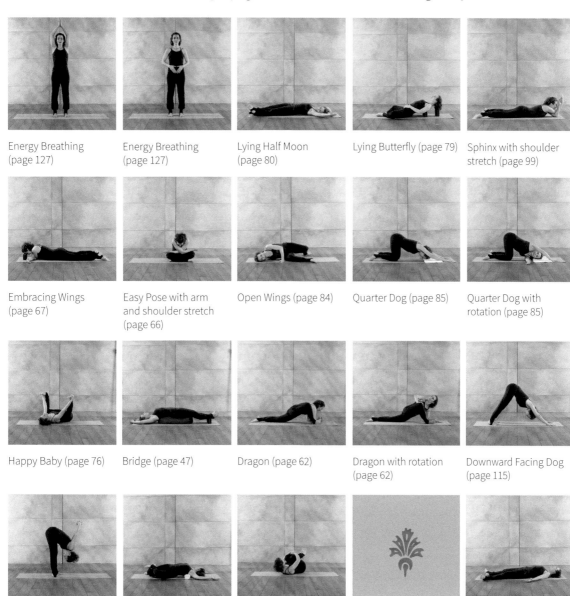

Energy Breathing
(page 127)

Energy Breathing
(page 127)

Lying Half Moon
(page 80)

Lying Butterfly (page 79)

Sphinx with shoulder
stretch (page 99)

Embracing Wings
(page 67)

Easy Pose with arm
and shoulder stretch
(page 66)

Open Wings (page 84)

Quarter Dog (page 85)

Quarter Dog with
rotation (page 85)

Happy Baby (page 76)

Bridge (page 47)

Dragon (page 62)

Dragon with rotation
(page 62)

Downward Facing Dog
(page 115)

Standing Forward Bend
with arm stretch
(page 60)

Twisted Roots Heart
Opener (page 108)

Folded Pose (page 117)

Protective Meditation
(page 132)

Relaxed Supine Position
(page 87)

✤ Skin Problems

Our skin covers the entire body and defines our exterior, and therefore has a protective function. Skin changes are quickly visible to others, and many people are embarrassed about flaky or red skin or spots. Skin problems are on the increase. In alternative medicine, it is assumed that skin problems are also an expression of a disrupted detoxification. For this reason, the intestine plays a decisive role in therapy.

From a holistic perspective, the skin is the mirror of the soul. If you are emotionally sensitive, you often have sensitive skin, and if you are irritable then this often shows up in irritated skin. Things from within always want to be seen—and this comes out externally via the skin.

✤ Possible questions for reflection are:
What inside me would like to be seen, and what might I have suppressed?
How can I have better boundaries with things or people that stress me?
Can I deal with touch?

From the TCM perspective, the defensive Chi is weakened with skin problems, and therapy is always carried out on the lungs. However, as there are countless complaint patterns, other factors are considered as well:

- With genetic skin complaints, such as psoriasis, it is the kidney.
- With moist pustules and blisters, it is the liver and gallbladder.
- With constitutional weaknesses or poor nutrition, it is the spleen and stomach.
- With stress, it is the liver and large intestine.

✤ To detoxify the intestine as much as possible and keep it healthy in the long term, regular intestine-cleansing treatments, colon hydrotherapy, or enemas are recommended. A diet that is rich in fiber, and two to three liters of non-carbonated water and herbal tea every day, will support the functioning of the intestine. You can also strengthen the intestinal flora with probiotics—particularly (and in any case) after a cleansing treatment or taking antibiotics. Industrially manufactured food, meat, sausage, white flour products, and sugar can upset the healthy balance of the bacteria in the intestine and should therefore be taken off the menu if you want to treat skin problems. ✤

In addition to the **meridian massage** (page 36), I recommend this **Yin Yoga sequence:**

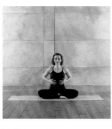

Full Breathing
(page 128)

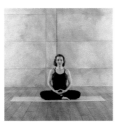

Ujjayi Breathing
(page 129)

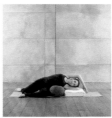

Lying Banana (page 78)

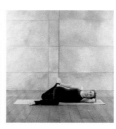

Cat Pulling Its Tail
(page 50)

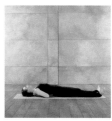

Twisted Arms (page 105)

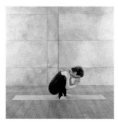

Squat (page 103)

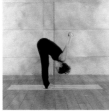

Standing Forward Bend
with arm stretch
(page 60)

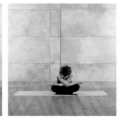

Easy Pose with arm
and shoulder stretch
(page 66)

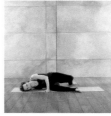

Open Wings (page 84)

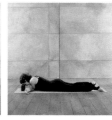

Embracing Wings
(page 105)

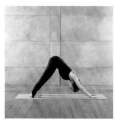

Downward Facing Dog
(page 115)

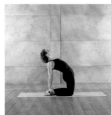

Camel (page 113)

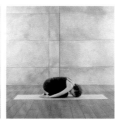

Child's Pose (page 57)

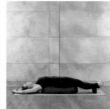

Bridge (page 47)

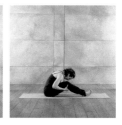

Coachman (page 51)

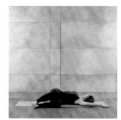

Twisted Roots
(page 106)

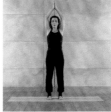

Energy Breathing
(page 127)

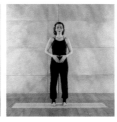

Energy Breathing
(page 127)

Protective Meditation
(page 132)

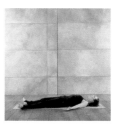

Relaxed Supine Position
(page 87)

❦ Susceptibility to Infections

By susceptibility to infections, we mean if the number of infections occurring is above average. For adults, about four infections per year is normal, and children usually succumb to infections more frequently, as their immune system cannot usually counter so many pathogens. Various pathogens can cause a variety of symptoms, but virus infections are most frequent and can lead to colds or stomach and intestine complaints. The causes of susceptibility to infections are many: besides lack of vitamins and minerals, environmental pollution, constant negative stress, inflammations, allergies, disrupted intestinal flora, lack of sleep, and too many stimulants or metabolic disorders may also be responsible.

From a holistic perspective, susceptibility to infections stands for a weakness of the immune system (at the physical level), as well as overstepping your own boundaries. There can also be a feeling of constant struggle and not being in the flow.

❧ **Possible questions for reflection are:**
What is taking up an unnecessarily large amount of energy in my life, and how can I avoid this?
What do I need to trust in the flow in my life again?
How can I better delimit the factors that do not do me any good?

From a TCM perspective, for a weakness in the defensive Chi function, lungs / large intestine, spleen / stomach, and kidneys / bladder are treated. To bring the general balance back into harmony and to stabilize it, however, the functioning of the liver and gallbladder, as well as the heart and small intestine, should also be included in the sequence.

> ❧ For susceptibility to infections, a diet that is nutritious and full of vitamins, with fresh and seasonal products, is recommended. Citrus fruits, kiwis, cabbage, and peppers supply abundant vitamin C, while dark green vegetables such as broccoli, savoy cabbage, spinach, and (wild) herbs score well with a high proportion of chlorophyll, another effective antioxidant. Fruits and vegetables also contain many secondary plant substances that have antiviral and antibacterial characteristics. Besides this, Omega-3 fatty acids, such as is found in linseed oil, for example, strengthen resistance. Also important for the immune system are foods rich in protein such as nuts, almonds and seeds (particularly hemp), whole-grain products (no wheat if you are gluten-sensitive, because it can even weaken the immune system), eggs, and legumes. ❧

In addition to the **meridian massage** (page 36), I recommend this **Yin Yoga sequence:**

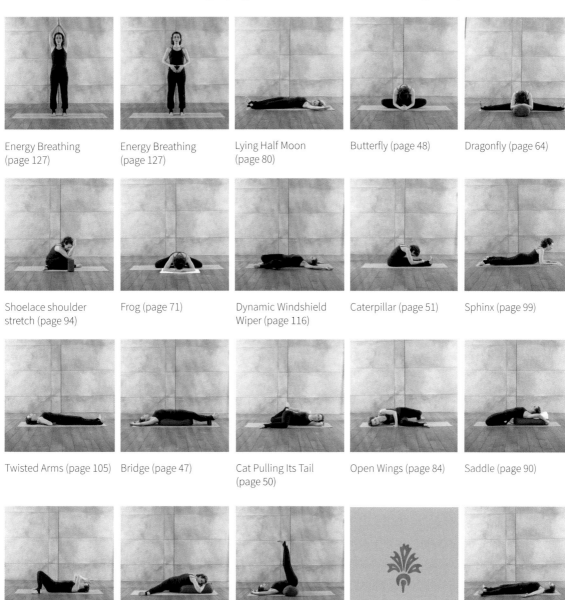

Energy Breathing
(page 127)

Energy Breathing
(page 127)

Lying Half Moon
(page 80)

Butterfly (page 48)

Dragonfly (page 64)

Shoelace shoulder
stretch (page 94)

Frog (page 71)

Dynamic Windshield
Wiper (page 116)

Caterpillar (page 51)

Sphinx (page 99)

Twisted Arms (page 105)

Bridge (page 47)

Cat Pulling Its Tail
(page 50)

Open Wings (page 84)

Saddle (page 90)

Resting Pose (page 89)

Sitting Twisted Roots
(page 96)

Seagrass (page 92)

Protective Meditation
(page 132)

Relaxed Supine
Position (page 87)

✤ Uncertainty and Indecision

Probably everyone is aware of their own tendencies towards uncertainty and indecision. Ultimately, there are decisions that have to be considered in detail—for example, a change of job or a move. Many things can be decided purely intuitively if we listen to our inner voice. But the mind often tries to intervene here. Intuition always reacts first; it is the first impulse that we feel when we address something. The mind only comes into it shortly afterwards. These are the moments when we feel uncertain and are torn between our inner voice and our mind. In some people, however, this uncertainty is particularly marked. They torture themselves when making a decision, and always need confirmation before they do so. Strong uncertainty can also be seen with addictions, depression, or anxiety disorders.

From a holistic perspective, marked indecision or a lack of self-assurance is associated with the loss of inner self-confidence. Contact has been lost with the inner voice, and you want to rely on the judgment of others so as not to make any mistakes. There may be a high level of perfectionism behind this, as well as anxiety about not gaining the recognition of others.

✤ Possible questions for reflection are:
Why am I worried about making decisions?
What is the worst that could happen if I make a wrong decision?
What do I have to do to be able to trust my inner voice again?

From a TCM perspective, indecision is a sign of a weak gallbladder. The liver, which forms a functional circuit with the gallbladder, stands for willingness to make decisions, while the gallbladder represents the courage to implement the decision.

> ✤ **If indecision is a major topic for you, then try to venture into making your own decisions in stages: trust your inner impulse. Try this first with small matters which do not have any great significance, and then keep aiming a little higher. Watch how it feels to have made a decision. You are sure to be rather proud of it, and you will trust yourself more often and more quickly to decide things all by yourself. ✤**

In addition to the **meridian massage** (page 36), I recommend this **Yin Yoga sequence:**

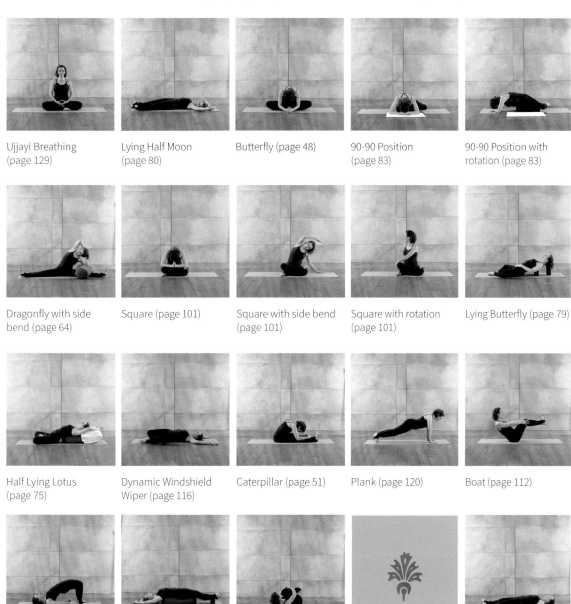

Ujjayi Breathing (page 129)

Lying Half Moon (page 80)

Butterfly (page 48)

90-90 Position (page 83)

90-90 Position with rotation (page 83)

Dragonfly with side bend (page 64)

Square (page 101)

Square with side bend (page 101)

Square with rotation (page 101)

Lying Butterfly (page 79)

Half Lying Lotus (page 75)

Dynamic Windshield Wiper (page 116)

Caterpillar (page 51)

Plank (page 120)

Boat (page 112)

Active Bridge (page 111)

Bridge (page 47)

Folded Pose (page 117)

Stillness Meditation (page 132)

Relaxed Supine Position (page 87)

❧ Worries, Brooding, Sadness, and Grief

Many people worry about things that will never happen. They make their own life difficult through their thoughts and unnecessary brooding. Sadness and grief, on the other hand, usually have a real and tangible cause, and they are not negative emotions, although they are often understood as such. Grief is very painful and it is therefore oftentimes suppressed. Nevertheless, it is an immensely important emotion which must be accepted and worked through so that it can be healed. If feelings such as worry or grief are too overwhelming, it can be very helpful to work through them with a therapist.

From a holistic perspective, considerable worry stands for a lack of basic trust. It is important to always ground yourself and regain trust. Yin Yoga has a very grounding effect, as most positions are carried out on the floor. Generally it is good to sit on the floor or spend as much time as possible in nature. Also, walking barefoot a lot or gardening can help to ground yourself.

❧ Possible questions for reflection are:

Why has my basic trust become weakened, and how can I develop more trust?
Can I recognize that many past worries were completely unnecessary?
What do I have to do in order to be able to let go better?
How do I regain access to my inner sources of strength?

In TCM, people who worry a great deal or brood have treatment for their spleen. The spleen is the mother of all organs and nourishes the entire body. The lungs can be treated, too, as they are associated with the emotions of sadness and grief. At a physical level, the spleen transports energy to the lungs to connect it with the energy of the breath there, and this paired energy is distributed throughout the whole body.

> ❧ If you experience emotions that make you uncomfortable, it is easy to resort to stimulants such as alcohol and sweets to comfort the mind. This is a fallacy, of course, as the effect only lasts for a short time, and ultimately the situation worsens. At such moments, try to find another form of balance. It often helps to talk to a good friend, take time in nature, or do a yoga practice. Moreover, the same nutrition recommendations apply as for the topic of anxieties (see page 142). ❧

In addition to the **meridian massage** (page 36), I recommend this **Yin Yoga sequence:**

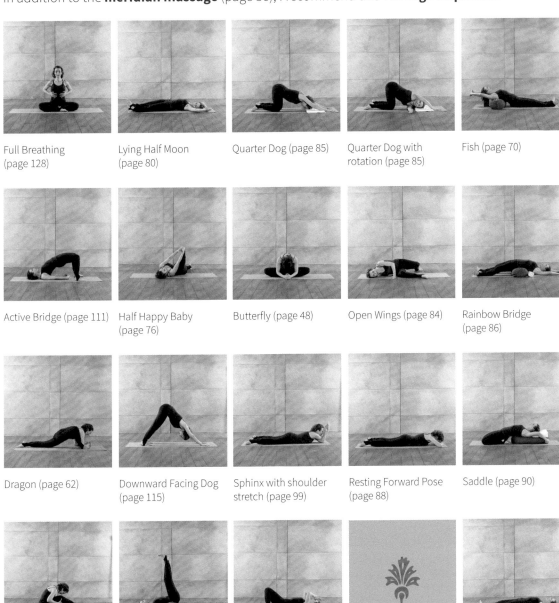

Full Breathing
(page 128)

Lying Half Moon
(page 80)

Quarter Dog (page 85)

Quarter Dog with
rotation (page 85)

Fish (page 70)

Active Bridge (page 111)

Half Happy Baby
(page 76)

Butterfly (page 48)

Open Wings (page 84)

Rainbow Bridge
(page 86)

Dragon (page 62)

Downward Facing Dog
(page 115)

Sphinx with shoulder
stretch (page 99)

Resting Forward Pose
(page 88)

Saddle (page 90)

Coachman (page 51)

Seagrass (page 92)

Resting Pose (page 89)

Protective Meditation
(page 132)

Relaxed Supine Position
(page 87)

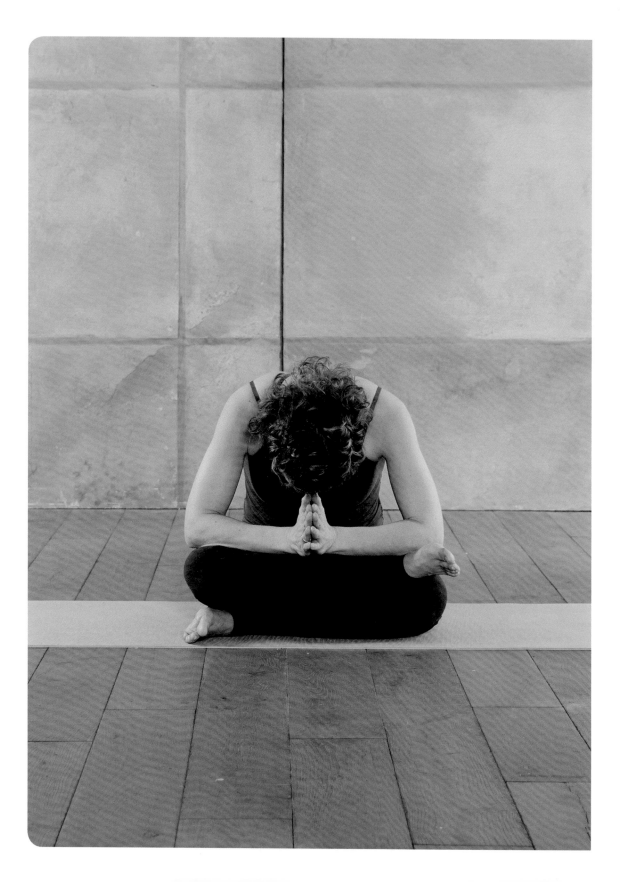

❦ Afterword

Thank you for taking the time to read this book and thereby letting me accompany you on your journey. I have given you a range of options with which I personally have had good experiences. But none of it is set in stone. You can only discover your own truth for yourself. I would like to encourage you to question things and find out for yourself whether they suit you as well as they do other people. If that is not the case, then you should respect the uniqueness of your body and find your own ways. Learn to treat yourself with empathy, love, and respect. Take responsibility for yourself, use your own wisdom in doing so, and trust your body. I wish you many blessings on your way!

❦ **OM MANI PADME HUM** ❦

❧ Acknowledgments

I would like to give my warmest thanks to my beloved family, who always support me in making my books and projects a reality. I wish to thank my teachers, who have shared their valuable knowledge with me—above all Paul and Suzee Grilley, but also all the people who have supported me on my yoga path so far. Their open and constant feedback gives me the opportunity to always continue learning. A big thank you to Dr. Angela Montenegro, who listened and responded patiently while I was drafting these sequences and answered any questions on the background of TCM. I would like to thank the entire team at She Writes Press, as well as Suedwest Verlag in Germany, where I first published this book. I also thank the photographers Lisa Martin and Renate Forster for their great cooperation, which has been a delight and a lot of fun. Thank you to Mary Barbosa for patiently proofreading this book over and over again and to Eileen Duhné for helping me bring it out into the world. All of you are a gift in my life. I thank the Universe for all the blessings, wonder, and love that I experience anew each day.

Namasté, love and light,

Stefanie Arend

❦ Index

❦ Selected Titles from **She Writes Press**

She Writes Press is an independent publishing company founded to serve women writers everywhere. Visit us at www.shewritespress.com.

Braided: A Journey of a Thousand Challahs by Beth Ricanati, MD. $16.95, 978-1-63152-441-7. What if you could bake bread once a week, every week? What if the smell of fresh bread could turn your house into a home? And what if the act of making the bread—mixing and kneading, watching and waiting—could heal your heartache and your emptiness, your sense of being overwhelmed? It can.

The Self-Care Solution: A Modern Mother's Must-Have Guide to Health and Well-Being by Julie Burton. $16.95, 978-1-63152-068-6. Full of essential physical, emotional and relational self-care tools—and based on research by the author that includes a survey of hundreds of moms—this book is a life raft for moms who often feel like they are drowning in the sea of motherhood.

The Art of Play: Igniting Your Imagination to Unlock Insight, Healing, and Joy by Joan Stanford. $19.95, 978-1-63152-030-3. Lifelong "non-artist" Joan Stanford shares the creative process that led her to insight and healing, and shares ways for others to do the same.

The Vitamin Solution: Two Doctors Clear the Confusion about Vitamins and Your Health by Dr. Romy Block and Dr. Arielle Levitan. $17.95, 978-1-63152-014-3. Drs. Romy Block and Arielle Levitan cut through all of the conflicting data about vitamins to provide readers with a concise, medically sound approach to vitamin use as a means of feeling better and enhancing health.

Raw by Bella Mahaya Carter. $16.95, 978-1-63152-345-8. In an effort to holistically cure her chronic stomach problems, Bella Mahaya Carter adopted a 100 percent raw, vegan diet—a first step on a quest that ultimately dragged her, kicking and screaming, into spiritual adulthood.

Painting Life: My Creative Journey Through Trauma by Carol K. Walsh. $16.95, 978-1-63152-099-0. Carol Walsh was a psychotherapist working with traumatized clients when she encountered her own traumatic experience; this is the story of how she used creativity and artistic expression to heal, recreate her life, and ultimately thrive.